I0623366

THE OPTIMISTICS

Richie Frieman

The Omnibus Publishing
Baltimore, MD

The Optimistics by Richie Frieman
1. Biography and Autobiography: Memoir 2. Health & Fitness: Diseases & Conditions: Alzheimer's & Dementia 3. Family & Relationships: Friendships

ISBN: 979-8-9854108-8-4

Library of Congress Control Number: 2024938143

Cover design by Richie Frieman and The Omnibus Publishing
Edited by Wendy Dean, MAE

Printed in the United States of America

The Omnibus Publishing is a division of Reading Pandas, Inc. Please send all written queries to the address below

The Omnibus Publishing
Attn: Non-fiction Editor's Desk
5422 Ebenezer Rd.
PO Box 152
White Marsh, MD 21162

Special Notes: (1) YES!, Inc. (Young-onset dementia Education & Support) is a 501(c)(3) organization, established to address the under recognized and growing needs of the YOD (Young-Onset Dementia) community. The author has removed the "!" throughout the text to avoid confusion with punctuation and improve the flow of text for the reader. (2) Young-Onset Dementia is capitalized by the medical community when written out; however, the "Y" in YES!, Inc. stands for Young-onset dementia and is not capitalized by the organization as part of their business name.

Contents

The Optimistics Mantra...10

Introduction...12

Chapter 1: Bubbe—The Duchess of Duckpin........................17

Chapter 2: The Walk...24

Chapter 3: Jim—Mr. Lighthouse 30

Chapter 4: Dennis—Time is Important................................43

Chapter 5: Mike—Our General Washington.........................63

Chapter 6: Karla and Michael—The Girl From Manaus.......76

Chapter 7: Dave and Kathy—Hello, Gorgeous.....................96

Chapter 8: Mark and Evie—Evie and the Frozen
   Orange...106

Chapter 9: Katherine and Sarah—Hugging Cows and Other
   Dreams..122

Chapter 10: Debbie and Shannon—The House That Shannon
   Built..135

Chapter 11: Donna and Alisha—X-It to Exit.......................155

Chapter 12: Shara and Audra—3AM Dreams......................167

Chapter 13: Chris and Linda—Life in a Fish Bowl...............177

Chapter 14: Glen and Val—The Singer and the Song...........184

Chapter 15: Lorinn—A Bicycle in the Shower......................198

Chapter 16: Andy and Laurie—Baseball, Bruce, and

   Traveling...210

Chapter 17: Daniel and Lisa—Watch with Wonder...........226

Chapter 18: Wendy and Doug—Midnight Journal................242

Chapter 19: Looking Back and Walking Forward...................256

Thank You..263

Resources and Support..264

About the Author...271

To Mike, Jim, and Dennis, who showed me what it means to be an Optimistic, and never forget that time is important.

"I put my hand in yours, and together we can do what we could never do alone."

—Mike, The Optimistics

The Optimistics' Mantra

A quick note about how the Optimistics' mantra came to be for the group. During a monthly Alzheimer's Association support group meeting attended by over thirty people living with Alzheimer's Dementia and their care partners, Mike kindly interrupted to make an announcement.

"Before we begin, can you please hold hands with the person next to you and repeat the Optimistics' mantra with me?"

Everyone in the room was happy to do so and followed along with him. Comments like, "Mike, that was so sweet," and, "Mike, that's very kind of you," echoed throughout the room afterward.

The next day while having coffee with Mike and Dennis, I asked, "How did you come up with such a compassionate mantra, Mike?"

He took a sip of coffee, then said, "I stole it."

"Stole it?"

"Well, I tweaked it," he corrected.

"From who?"

In a typical, nonchalant, and soft spoken Mike-manner, he replied, "Overeaters Anonymous."

Immediately I started laughing. Dennis and Mike joined in and soon tears fell from my eyes.

"Is that wrong?" Mike asked me, still laughing at himself.

"Well, it's not ours, bud, so kinda, yeah."

"Do you think they'll know?"

"Who? Overeaters Anonymous?"

"Yeah."

"Let's hope they never search our website and then we're safe."

We couldn't control ourselves from that moment.

"It does fit us though," said Dennis.

"No argument there. But I say we work on a new one," I recommended.

Mike thought for a moment. "Okay, but it's still a good one for now."

"Yes, yes it certainly works well for now, Mike."

To this day, Mike, Dennis, and I still think about that conversation and laugh. It's one of the little moments with the Optimistics that remind me of how they changed my life. I'd also learn that a day like that was just another day at the office for me and the Optimistics.

Introduction

Nobody wanted this book. Not publishers, not agents, not editors—no one.

Why is that? Quoting one rather obtuse publisher, "People are scared to talk about Alzheimer's, let alone when it affects young adults buying the book."

Another publisher saw my vision and wanted to add *The Optimistics* to their catalog as a 2026 release. I told them that we didn't have that much time and that I needed this book to be out sooner. Well, not to ruin the punchline, but guess how that turned out?

One agent told me, "Who wants to read about Alzheimer's while they are lying on a beach?"

Great. Thanks. I'm glad to know where the bar is set.

Then again, who am I to argue what the industry deems "ideal" for publishing? I'm just some writer with keyboard-scabbed fingertips and a bizarre belief that people could use a heavy dose of hope in their lives. But that's me being me. These publishers are the real professionals.

I guess I could have turned the Optimistics a superhero graphic novel. Giving characters their secret identities while trying to manage a deadly condition by day and fight crime by night. Wait! How about a "Who Done It?" mystery filled with cliff-hanging suspense to set up for the sequel? Better yet, let's make the Optimistics a ragtag group of friends bitten by a pack of vampires who spend eternity hunting their prey. People love vampires! Those ideas would fly off the shelves, and just in time for the summer reading buzz.

Despite the industry's intolerance to discuss something "as negative as Alzheimer's," the nuances of the literary world did have one thing right: all forms of dementia are scary. I discuss uncomfortable topics which are a given with Alzheimer's Dementia and Related Dementias (ADRD), but it's not this book's purpose. The story of the Optimistics is about family, hope, love, and compassion. It's also filled with romantic unities between couples that surpass every poetic wedding vow ever spoken. Although ADRD are frightening, the founders of the Optimistics, Dennis, Mike, and Jim, created a cultural movement in understanding how to live life with an incurable condition through their positivity.

In this book, you'll hear me repeat words like hope, optimism, love, time, moments, connection, and commitment. All these have become undeniable trends in the lives of the Optimistics. I'll also discuss fear and "the darkness," a term that every care partner and individual with dementia uses to describe the hole this disease creates for all parties involved. Despite the impact of fear, you will also discover how everyone found a way to crawl out of the darkness and into the light. So, if you can't handle a glimpse of reality and a mature topic like this, one that shows how support and empathy will always win over fear, this book isn't for you.

I'll pause to allow anyone with blinders to exit the stage left while the rest of us continue.

Despite the rejections I received for this book, I couldn't waste time yelling at my ceiling in frustration. Granted, I did spend hours giving the middle finger to my inbox, but if there's one thing I've learned about ADRD, it's that giving up is a terrible use of time. As the oldest Optimistic, Dennis, told me in an email, "Time is important."

Time is important.

I repeated that phrase throughout writing this book, scribbled it on paper, taped that saying to my desk, and continued telling myself time is important until the last word was written. Time is not only critical in the lives of the Optimistics but also limited. The Optimistics are all aware that their clock is winding down rapidly. With the effects of ADRD chipping away at the lives of millions of people with these diseases each day, both physically and mentally, I knew that regardless of how fast I worked, the Optimistics themselves may not be able to enjoy this book properly. Some would not even be around to read it.

Young-Onset Dementia (YOD) affects the behavior and cognition of people younger than sixty-five years old. This is what connects the Optimistics. Those with YOD lose memories by the day at a speed that no one can govern. Making peace with that understanding allowed me to realize a more profound mission. Quickly, the Optimistics moved from strangers to best friends who weren't afraid to cry in front of one another. Through their bond, they understood the desire for compassion around ADRD is not limited to the original three Optimistics. The mission of the Optimistics has grown to embrace others in similar scenarios. The Optimistics' story wasn't solely for Dennis, Mike, and Jim; it was for the dozens of families across the country in the YOD community whom I met with similar stories.

The more I got involved in the Optimistics' world, the more profound their message became. I met Deb and Evie, who are two of the founders of the YES Program (Young-Onset Dementia Education and Support); a support group catering to individuals, family members, and care partners living with YOD. From there, I met Shannon, a lawyer who was inspired by her mother's dementia to navigate her legal career in elder care law. I also met Sarah, who, at only twenty-three, became her mother's legal guardian, all while in college. Then there was Lorrin, Val, Glenn, Daniel, Audra, Shannon, Sarah, Alisha, Laurie, Doug, Michael, Kathy, and many others—all of whom proudly call themselves Optimistics.

In each new conversation, I gained a deeper perspective into a community that brought me tears of sadness and of joy. Together we talked about fear, loss, compassion, and, of course, optimism. As I uncovered more about each member of the Optimistics community, I learned more about myself, which stirred up new questions about who I am and who I want to become.

—How can I handle hard times that seem too much to bear?

—How can I be a better parent when there's too much out of my control?

—How can I be a better spouse and build a better future for my wife?

—How do I manage the ups and downs of a career and a timetable I only see?

—How do I not throw the towel in when I feel lost?

What I thought would be a memoir about three men and their personal battles turned into an international outreach campaign to share the message of people whose stories will change the lives of many. Thankfully, I realized I wasn't alone in my views. The idea of ADRD is scary, let alone having to cope with dementia in your 30s, 40s, or 50s when your life and career are beginning to hit their glory days. Having to accept how this diagnosis changed their lives so early in the aging process, the Optimistics proved that dementia spares no one. However, that doesn't mean you're alone.

The Optimistics have provided each other with a torch of humanity to combat the shadows appearing in the loneliest times. Together, they've spotlighted dementia and found a much needed boost as a united team rather than living in isolation. Through the support of each other, they also discovered that life doesn't stop at a diagnosis.

Alas, there may not be any caped crusaders in this book, but I promise you there are heroes. The Optimistics showed me a new way to try for a better version of myself and everyone I met along the way. They also taught me the power of time and how to prioritize what's most important in your life so each day is more valuable than the last. They showed me that with love and support, you can drive past the agony this disease brings at speeds faster than you ever imagined while the wind wipes your tears away before they have a chance to fall from your cheeks. Most importantly, they allowed me solace to see that regardless of the hazardous roads ahead, there will always be someone by your side along life's unpredictable journey.

It's in those feelings you will find eternal optimism.

CHAPTER ONE

BUBBE

THE DUCHESS OF DUCKPIN

I remember the blank stares and wailing. I must have been around nine or ten when it first started. My Bubbe, Sophie, was a stocky brick of iron but with a tender heart and an even sweeter smile. When I was in kindergarten, she used to take me Duckpin bowling during her weekend leagues in Baltimore. At only 4'10", she could throw the ball down the lane with the force of a shot putter and could curve a bowling ball so sharply it would make David Beckham jealous. Her bowling friends and members of the Ladies Hi Game Club, as their team shirts read, would grab my chubby cheeks while I stuffed my mouth with French fries.

Even though I enjoyed the fine cuisine of a bowling alley in the early 80s, what I liked most about my bowling trips with Bubbe was watching her win many trophies. She would let me have it, and being six, it was a big deal. What kid wouldn't want a shiny trophy to hold onto, even if it was of a woman in a skirt carrying a bowling ball? I didn't care. She handed them to me and made me feel like a winner.

At the time, I didn't realize my family dynamic. My parents had divorced before any memory of them together. On the weekends, my brother and I would sleep at my dad's house. I didn't know that my dad's house at that time was my grandparents' while he transitioned after the divorce. But none of that seemed weird to me—I loved it. On Friday nights, we'd have Shabbat dinner, with Bubbe cooking the most mouth-watering corned beef and matzo ball soup I'd ever tasted. After that, my dad, brother, and I would walk from their house to The Reisterstown Road Plaza, where we'd pick out something from Kay-B-Toys. As fun as the toy store was, Saturdays were the real gift.

Every Saturday morning, I'd wake up to find Bubbe and Grandpa in the living room. Grandpa wore his standard attire of a white button-up and black slacks, smoking cigarettes in his recliner. He'd always sneak me a shiny green rectangle of Andes Chocolate Mints, which he kept in a glass bowl beside his ashtray. Bubbe was always in a day dress of some sort, either preparing a meal or in her chair as they watched TV. When I came down, though, Bubbe had to watch what I wanted—professional wrestling.

Back in the 80s, there were different professional wrestling shows on Saturday mornings, and Bubbe and I would watch them for hours together in the living room. While I was dreaming of becoming a professional wrestler one day, Bubbe would tease me by saying it was fake and that the wrestlers were idiots. Still, she humored me as we cheered on my in-ring idols and booed the heels.

Bowling, food, and professional wrestling were the first images I had of my grandmother; however, the final memories of Bubbe weren't as pleasant. Not only did Bubbe have Alzheimer's Dementia (AD), but she also overcame breast cancer somewhere along the way. I recall the cancer being hidden from me, but AD was something that could not go unnoticed. The years between the fun-filled weekends at my grandparents and the deterioration of Bubbe because of dementia come in waves to this day. Highlights of my time with Bubbe flow across my memory like buoys, guiding me along my journey to understand this disease. With AD, memories of the past are what hold together the future, not only for those affected by dementia but their loved ones. Like Bubbe's changes throughout her illness, the lives around family and friends must also move forward.

When I was around eight, my dad moved out of my grandparents' house and in with a longtime girlfriend. We would still eat Shabbat dinner and continue the Saturday morning visits. Over time, piece by piece, the routine I became so accustomed to changed. First, Shabbat dinners stopped, then our Saturday visits became shorter and more infrequent. When we'd visit, Grandpa would sit in his front porch rocking chair with the paper with a wide smile and candy for me. Sometimes, we wouldn't even go inside because "Bubbe was sleeping," and hang out on the porch together for a half hour or so.

One Saturday morning, I learned why things were no longer the same. Inside their house, my grandparents' bed replaced the dining room table. Grandpa's recliner was out of the living room and now next to Bubbe as she rested under blankets. I implied the move was because of arthritis in Bubbe's leg, which made sense. She could hardly walk any longer, let alone handle the narrow stairs. I'd kiss her hello, we'd talk, Grandpa would slip me some candy as always, and then Dad and I would go to a movie before being dropped off at my mom's house. Those were my weekend routines with Dad until dementia took complete control of Bubbe's body.

That was when I first saw dementia in action.

My first recollection of Bubbe's Alzheimer's—and Alzheimer's Dementia in general—was her eyes. When I'd come over, I'd still kiss her on her cheek, but now her majestic ocean eyes were watered as if she had been crying for hours. It's likely she was. She'd cup my face and say, "I love you, Richard. I love you!"

I can still feel the touch of her chubby, cold hands on my face.

Her eyes would dance around at me as if looking for answers in my face.

Then she'd start to cry.

When I was around eleven or twelve, Bubbe had already been crying in agony long before we even got to her house. She was in so much pain from her leg that she would scream for my grandfather to cut it off.

"Al just put it in the window and slam it down shut. Get rid of it, Al!"

Grandpa would try to defuse the awkwardness with a joke by saying, "Okay, Sophie, I'll do that later. Maybe after lunch."

Then he'd wink at me as if to say that Bubbe was being silly. Despite that humor, even though I had no idea what dementia was by definition, I knew Bubbe's personality change was due to something other than her leg.

On some visits, when I went down to kiss her hello, she would look me in the eyes and say, "I'm so happy to see you, Ben."

Ben was her brother, who had passed away decades ago.

Dad would correct her. "That's not Ben, Mom. That's Richie." She'd look at the ceiling and roll her head side to side, wailing, "Richard? Oh, I love you, Richie."

Then she'd cry.

"Love you too, Bubbe."

I remember trying to contain my emotions in front of my dad because I wanted to keep those Saturday morning visits going as long as possible. Then there was the last visit to their house that I can recall. I was around thirteen, right after my Bar Mitzvah. When we arrived, Bubbe was yelling at my grandfather about something nonsensical. Dad walked me in and I hugged Grandpa, then kissed Bubbe.

"It's Richie, Mom," Dad said.

"Oh, Richard. Richard," she said, holding my face. "Richard."

Dad and I sat in the dining room around Bubbe, talking to Grandpa. Bubbe would go in and out of moaning and mumbling. Then, she said, "Richard, I'll be at your Bar Mitzvah."

We had talked about my Bar Mitzvah at every visit, and I knew how important it was to her.

"Mom, we already had Richie's Bar Mitzvah," Dad reminded her.

"What?! Where was I?"

"You couldn't come, Mom. It's okay, Dad was there."

"Al? Ben?" she cried.

"No, Mom, Uncle Ben died a long time ago."

Then she cried out more, but rather than sadness, it was anger, confusion, frustration, and guilt.

"Richard, I'm so sorry I wasn't there! I wanted to be there!"

"I know, Bubbe. It's okay," I'd reminded her.

That is the last memory I have of Bubbe inside my grandparents' house.

Bubbe's condition developed too intensely for my grandfather to manage at his age as well as his own health. To help with her care, she was put into a nursing home not far from their house. Despite being in a home, Dad still took me to see Bubbe every Saturday before our movie. I can picture every square inch of that nursing home, which still brings me chills today. The second you got off the elevator, an intense stench of urine would waft through the air. The elderly roamed around like zombies, reaching for nurses and other visitors as they walked by. The front staff were doing less than the bare minimum and their attitudes were stronger than the awful smell of human waste.

By that time, even though she was there physically, the vicious claws of dementia had taken a full grasp of Bubbe's mind and body. At the nursing home, our visits were quick but meaningful. Although Bubbe had no idea who anyone was by this point, my dad still wanted me to see her, and I could never thank him enough for that experience. It was not easy, yet it was my dad's way of reminding me how important family is, regardless of the situation. He wasn't pretending she would get better; however, he showed me that being there for a loved one is what matters most.

Until her last breath, we would visit.

Sadly, I would find in writing this book that not everyone with dementia has the same support that Bubbe did. Mentioned in nearly every conversation was how some family members disappear after an Alzheimer's Dementia diagnosis because they don't know how to react to someone with the disease. The dejection flows in the heart of every care partner and spouse who has yet another reason to feel isolated.

My time with Bubbe left many impressions on me, but the biggest was that I can never be too frightened to say goodbye before it's too late. Time—as Dennis reminded me—is important. Yet being young and energetic, it never dawned on me until I met the Optimistics that dementia doesn't solely strike the elderly. That concept fueled my desire to pursue answers and stories from the Optimistics to find peace in the unknown that the future holds.

CHAPTER TWO

The Walk

"These guys are like the mortar between the bricks that keep us bonded when we're going through the hard times."
—Mike, The Optimistics

As a writer, people often ask me where I find inspiration. The answer is always the same. "Inspiration is all around, as long as you look for it," which, as I say each time, I realize it sounds cliché. Having written several books and hundreds of articles over the years, every project I worked on has been instigated by a particular event I have witnessed, which then parked itself into my brain. From there, the next step in my creative process involves developing a document with notes and ideas to consider whether the concept is something I'll pursue further. Some ideas stick harder than others. At the Walk to End Alzheimer's on October 22, 2022, in Hunt Valley, Maryland, I witnessed inspiration that became lodged in my soul.

I pulled into the jam-packed parking lot of the shopping center for the Walk on a chilly fall day with a coffee in hand. I was meeting one of my best friends, Geoff, who organized a team in honor of his late father, Arnie. The plan was to walk with Arnie, but a few months prior, Arnie passed away due to Alzheimer's Dementia (AD) and COVID-19 after being placed in a nursing home. Now this walk took on much more significance for our team. Open parking spots were hard to find between the thousands in attendance and a classic car show in the same shopping center. Yet, of all the spaces left open, in all the lanes I pulled down, I found one open space beside a bright yellow Corvette.

That usually wouldn't register as odd with me on any other occasion, but that day it hit me: Arnie drove the exact bright yellow Corvette. Despite the presence of thousands of cars, there was only one yellow Corvette. Arnie's yellow Corvette was so important to him that, for the Walk, Geoff's mom made our team yellow T-shirts with Arnie's face printed on them.

What were the chances? Nice one, Arnie.

I mentioned the car to Geoff when I finally met him by the Walk's entrance. He also saw it, which made him and his mom, Sheila, even more emotional for the day. The event was packed with families who all went through something similar, and each had their own story. There were spouses, children, grandchildren, volunteers, doctors, and people currently fighting dementia. I came to support Geoff, my Bubbe, and my wife's grandmother, Charlotte, whom I adored.

Geoff's family had a squad of supporters wearing yellow shirts in honor of Arnie, including Geoff's kids, extended family, and a few close friends. Geoff also brought his adorable Newfoundland puppy, Dierks. At 135 pounds of drool and gentleness, he attracted a lot of attention, which gave some lighthearted entertainment to the day. Before the walk began, there was an opening ceremony with a special guest speaker, Dennis Myers. Dennis was a physician's assistant who had stopped practicing medicine a few years prior due to his Young Onset Dementia (YOD) diagnosis. Geoff and his mom gasped when Dennis and his wife took the microphone.

"That's Dennis!" Sheila shouted.

"Who is Dennis?" I asked.

"Oh man, that's my dad's care provider. He was mine too when I was younger, until he had to stop because of his Alzheimer's." Geoff handed me Dierks's leash. "Watch him for a second. We're going to get closer."

They inched towards the stage while Dierks and I watched with the crowd. Dennis spoke eloquently about how he dealt with the disease. He talked about the support of his family, his excellent medical staff, the Alzheimer's Association, and especially the bond he created with an inspiring group of friends, Mike and Jim. The three friends nicknamed themselves the Optimistics, all diagnosed with YOD. The Optimistics made a pact to be with one another throughout their battles and share what they're going through and what they've learned. They also promised to lean on one another like family. The more time the Optimistics spent together, the more they became a unique sounding board of support as the only ones who could truly understand the magnitude of what each was going through. Hearing of their bond set a wave of emotion throughout the crowd. I could hear others around me happily murmur the same thing, "The Optimistics? That's a cool name."

I wasn't sure if I heard that right either. The name alone was an ironic punchline to an awful disease associated with any word but optimism. I listened to Dennis's story as his wife stood beside him the entire time, watching his face as he spoke and holding his arm in encouragement. The Optimistics were more than a group of friends bound by dementia. They had created a strategy for their friends and family to adopt, making each day a little easier. After all, if Dennis, Mike, and Jim can stay optimistic about their battle, surely those around them can also try—they hope.

After a round of applause, Dennis left the stage. Within seconds, Geoff and his mom approached him. They hugged Dennis and shook hands. When Geoff and Sheila came back to our group it was clear that seeing Dennis had brought out new emotions.

"He's such a sweet man," Sheila said in a crackled voice while dabbing her eyes with a tissue.

"How long have you known him?" I asked Geoff.

Geoff's dark eyes, surrounded by freckles, had been rubbed raw over the past several months, and today didn't help. His deep voice sounds like a mix between an old-school country singer and a voice actor who does movie trailers. He is a quiet guy, but he always sounds thoughtful when he talks.

He said, "I've known Dennis since I was a teenager. He helped me with all kinds of crap I had going on. He was also there for my dad since day one."

As best friends, Geoff and I have confided in one another for decades; however, that day introduced a new world of feelings I couldn't have anticipated. Geoff told me the night before the walk, "My dad was supposed to be here. When

I planned this walk months ago, I thought I was jinxing us because I was nervous something might happen before the Walk."

Geoff watched as other people approached Dennis while his sons, Gregory, 13, and Hudson, 9, joined his side to begin the walk. Geoff remained still and focused on Dennis. "He was the best care provider we ever had," Geoff said, scratching his five o'clock shadow.

"That's amazing, bud. I'm sure he was happy to see you."

"He didn't remember us," Geoff said in a deep voice to cover the knot in his throat. He adjusted his weathered Red Sox hat and added, "This disease, man, it robs people of everything. It robbed my dad and took away Dennis's career early. He spent his whole life helping people, and then this. This is what he gets? It's not fair."

As we began the Walk, I couldn't stop thinking about what Dennis talked about in his speech.

"Dennis said that he has a group called the Optimistics, right?" I asked.

A grin came out from the side of Geoff's mouth. "Yeah, can you believe it? He and some guys he met got together to be there for one another. It's incredible."

I nodded in agreement. "Incredible, to put it mildly."

We continued walking, distracting ourselves with good conversation and laughter as Dierks wobbled through the bushes rather than taking the sidewalk. Packs of people took photos with one another in their team shirts, waving Alzheimer's Association flowered windmills and soaking in the moment. Everyone was there for different reasons, but also for the same reason, and all were united with one another. While I thought about Bubbe and Charlotte, I couldn't stop thinking about the Optimistics.

Following my creative process, I took note of their group and tucked it away for the time being. However, unlike all the dozens and dozens of other ideas that will only ever live on my desktop, the Optimistics was one story I could not shake, even weeks after the event.

Whether it was a calling or a sign, I was hooked. I became obsessed with optimism and consumed with how someone in their situation would never give up.

Even though I was eager to hear more about the Optimistics, and possibly share their story with readers, familiar questions of self-doubt overshadowed my optimism.

—*Where do I even start?*

—*How do I reach out to strangers living with dementia and ask to be let into their lives?*

—*Would and should they allow me into their lives?*

—*Would they let me tell their story?*

—*What if I let them down?*

The last question scared me the most, but I couldn't let this idea slip away.

CHAPTER THREE

Jim

MR. LIGHTHOUSE

"Be kind, loving, and don't be an asshole. I **do not** raise assholes."

That was the first thing Jim's oldest child, Meaghan, told me when I asked what her father was like growing up. Jim said all three of his kids the same thing, and I can tell you firsthand that Jim did not raise assholes. Having met Jim many times over the past year and a half, I cannot imagine him ever cursing let alone living by such a colorful mantra. However, Meaghan and I know different versions of Jim. Listening to her and Jim's wife, Terri, talk about "Jim of the past," gave me a wild new vision of the one I speak to. It made me love him even more. I will never know who Jim was before his diagnosis, but what I know now is enough to see why he was always admired personally and professionally.

James, Jim, Jimmy, or Dad as he is known, always stood out. Being 6'5" and built like an NFL tight end, Jim makes an immediate impression when he enters a room, and it's been that way since he was a child. Always an athlete, he excelled at every sport thrown his way. Even if it were a sport Jim never tried, he would pick it up quickly, excel at it, and then make everyone else jealous. He excelled in high school football, basketball, and lacrosse. Then he took his basketball skills to the collegiate level. Terri tells me he was always the "Big Man on Campus," on and off the field. In the classroom, Jim was a math wizard, which later helped him with a career in finance and as a CFO for significant hospitals.

"Jim was always really well-liked," Terri said, remembering a teenage Jim. "The teachers loved him. He was a kind guy, not at all arrogant or anything like that."

Attesting to Jim's reputation as Mr. Popular, Terri knew of him in high school, but their paths never crossed. She had different interests, is three years older, and their circles never mingled. Despite years as strangers, they met the summer Terri graduated from college after Jim finished his first year. Jim immediately fell for Terri. They dated for a long time, and despite a slight break up, which Jim admittedly regretted, they got back together during Jim's senior year of college. Then, their lives together as a team began.

Terri became a nurse and Jim entered the corporate world focusing on his financial background. Soon, Meaghan was born, then Ryan, and later, Devon, to round out the Hursey crew. Jim not only instilled in his children the rule of having good manners but also taught all his children how to be star athletes. He drove to practices, helped coach in various sports, and stood on the sidelines as a proud parent at as many games as possible. It turns out that parenting came as natural as dunking a basketball, and the Hursey kids recognize it through Jim's actions.

Jim was the first person I saw at my first YES group meeting in 2022. He took over the entire room with his sheer presence because he looked like someone in charge. If you were to do an image search for "CFO for a Fortune 500 Company," his picture could be in the lineup. I told Terri that when I first saw Jim, he looked like someone who walked off a golf course at a corporate event or the stage at a political speech. Jim stands in a pristine posture with his hands in his pockets, then bends his neck to talk to people and hug them. His hefty laugh travels through his entire body, and you can't help but smile. Jim also has an unnatural ability to work a room without even moving, easily drawing people to him.

At that first meeting, I walked over to Jim, shook his hand, and was in awe of the "Jim effect." It's an aura that helped him climb the corporate ladder, skipping over rungs with long-legged leaps. Terri and Meaghan credit Jim's diligence in his career, which garnered high praise from his colleagues even when he was forced into an early retirement at fifty-two. Terri told me about his final day as CFO for a major hospital outside Baltimore. An employee whom Jim oversaw and mentored walked him to his car and wept the entire time. He hugged Jim goodbye, and Jim wished him well, officially handing over the torch. His mentee and everyone in the hospital knew they lost a great leader. Jim's team couldn't understand seeing him end his career at an age when other C-suiters were getting started.

Meaghan knows better than anyone about Jim's career's importance to him. "There were two dads: work dad and home dad," she said. "He worked all the time and loved it. He always wore a nice suit, and was very polite and respected."

Then, Meaghan added, "But when he was home, he was so goofy."

Even though he worked hard to earn the respect of his peers, he let his funny side out when it came to the young patients in the hospital. He would dress up for holidays in costumes and visit the rooms of sick kids to make them laugh for the moment. Despite being the center of attention, Meaghan said Jim never had "guy friends" that she can recall. He did not have a connection with others like he does now with Dennis and Mike.

"I love watching him with the Optimistics because it's the first time he's had that kind of bond with other men on that level. I've never seen him so close to people, other than his late brother, Bill."

Bill was more than an older brother to Jim. He was Jim's support and had planned to be a care partner for Jim once he entered his battle with dementia. Bill passed away shortly after Jim's diagnosis and the loss of his brother shattered every part of him.

With tears, Terri told me about the day they learned about Bill. "Only a couple of things have brought my husband to his knees, and one was when we had to tell him that Bill had died."

Terri took a moment to collect herself. "Jim said, 'No! Not Bill! Bill was going to be with me through this.'"

Even though their bond was unbreakable towards the end of Bill's life, Jim was reluctant to tell his brother about his diagnosis. As a result, the space Jim put between himself and his brother by avoiding the topic created a rift in the family.

"Bill couldn't figure out what was going on. And I couldn't tell Bill because it was Jim's story to tell, not mine," Terri said. "But Jim was distancing himself from his brother at that time. We all saw it."

Jim gained the courage to talk to Bill, and his response was exactly as you'd imagine it to be between two brothers bound by more than blood. Terri said, "Finally, Jim told Bill, and Bill said, 'Jimmy, I'm here for you. We're going to get through this together.'"

Although their connection was natural as adults, their friendship wasn't as great as children. Terri laughed when talking about them growing up together. "It's funny. When they were little, they always fought. You know, there was that rivalry because Jim was such a good athlete and stuff like that. Bill was too, but..." she grinned. "Then, I think it was when I started dating Jim, and definitely when we got married, that they got closer and closer. I mean, we would vacation together all the time."

Hearing about Bill's death and witnessing how Jim interacted with the others in the support group, I know how important it is for Terri and the other care partners to keep the Optimistics together. Meaghan realized the unfortunate timing of the Optimistics' brotherly relationships, which developed towards the tail end of their lives. She wished Jim had met them all years ago, albeit for different reasons.

Meaghan wishes a lot for her father now.

"He's not my dad," Meaghan said flatly. "Not the dad that I knew."

Being the oldest gives Meaghan more years of experience with her dad than her siblings. However, Devin chalked up more hours than most, having traveled cross country from Maryland to Seattle on her way-too-tiny car with Jim riding shotgun. It's one thing to travel cross country and another to travel cross country with a 6'5" frame, your knees bent against the glove box for hours on end. But that's the kind of father Jim will always be, regardless of how the disease affects him.

Meaghan said, "He didn't complain once! They had a great time together. They talked about movies and music. He loves classic rock, like the Eagles and KISS. Every car ride involving my dad included classic rock. The family is taking him to a KISS concert. He remembers words to every song and has a memory for each song too."

"Jim was able to sing along?"

"Yeah, I know. I was surprised as well."

I asked Jim and Terri about the road trip. Terri was so happy that the two of them had that time together, allowing them to develop a much stronger relationship. She is impressed by how her three children have handled Jim's condition, especially since Jim may not be around for many more family celebrations. In a discussion with Terri, I heard for the first time how severe Jim's decline has been over the past year. In my interactions with Jim, I could tell that he was quieter each time we met, but I didn't think that was an alarming sign of his dementia. Although to me, Jim appeared comfortable, looking back now, I can see that his quietness was Jim becoming more reticent towards the group due to his dementia.

During their Christmas dinner together, with all the Hursey family members in attendance, Terri realized the sad fact about Jim's status. "We all know this is most likely our last fun meal together." Terri took a pause. Then her lips quivered as she said, "It will probably be our last Christmas with Jim."

I tried to keep myself from breaking down, but I couldn't.

This was the first and only time any care partner had discussed their spouse with a definitive timetable. There was always a notion of "we'll see," but never "this will be it," until now. At that moment, I realized how strong Terri and her children have been through Jim's illness. And, sooner than they envisioned, there would be an empty chair at every holiday where Jim used to sit.

"You don't think he'll make it that long?" I asked, hoping I heard her wrong.

"The rate that he's declining, Richie. I feel like, and I've said this in the group to the women and men, almost every three months, there will be a pretty sharp decline."

Again, I was unable to handle that news. He's Jim! He's this grand figure of a man and such a joyous presence, with a sunny demeanor that I can't envision leaving us all. I told Terri I was sorry. It was sincere, but it was the only thing I could manage.

She appreciated the gesture. Terri knows that, like me, everyone around Jim can't imagine his impressive presence being taken away from us so quickly. She added, "I could very well see this upcoming summer that I may have to place him somewhere. He's six foot five and 200 some-odd pounds, and there's only so much I will be able to do with him, you know? So, that's kind of what I'm thinking."

We matched eyes and I nodded with her. Terri allowed her emotions to flow freely, stating out loud the past several months have been particularly hard. "I don't know. I just don't know."

I have met other care partners who faced a similar excruciating decision of allowing a separate dwelling facility to care for a loved one. Terri admitted she can't help but feel guilty. Still, she knows it's the best option for Jim's care.

"I will never judge anyone for whatever decisions they choose to make because everyone has limits on what they can do. What if he falls? That's over 200 pounds I have to pick up."

I stressed that anyone in her position would do the same thing. "I mean, it's just from the fear of physicality. That's not your fault, Terri."

The pure reality of understanding one's strengths and abilities is a fact you can't ignore. Terri would be doing a disservice to Jim and her mental health to think otherwise. I can't help but hurt for Terri when trying to understand the unfair emotions that guilt brings in dark moments. I also believe that if Jim could express himself the way he could before the diagnosis, he would beg her to do the same thing. After all, the Jim I've gotten to know lived life with an analytical approach to problem-solving. One solution is the definitive answer to an issue based on research. Terri's abilities and Jim's severity are problems, and there is only one true option now.

Jim's career was about taking his heart out of a situation and only focusing on the numbers. Right now, there is no way to avoid the statistics of dementia or the realities of what

Terri is capable of at her age. With all the stresses of Jim's care weighing her down, Terri tries to focus on the now, what she can control, and finding joy in her time with Jim each day.

"What do you think Jim's mindset is on remaining optimistic and for all of you?"

"I think he can't even," she began, then stopped herself before finishing the thought. "What one person said to me about this disease is that the person with Alzheimer's can't realize what's happening to them. Jim looked at me one time, and he goes, 'It's not like I have a disease or anything,' and I decided okay, we'll go with that."

Meaghan said something similar about responding to Jim's fluctuating thought process. Once at their house, Jim pointed to a dog in their yard. Meaghan told me there was no dog. Yet, at that moment, she could either tell Jim he was wrong or go along. As Terri has done, Meaghan chose the latter. She told me it wasn't even worth debating. "Let him think there's a dog. Who cares? That's fine."

Along with the cognitive aspects of dementia's decline, Jim's speech has begun to diminish as well. Terri struggles to comprehend most of what Jim tells her and has to do her best to piece together his needs. "I can probably only understand maybe 30% to 40% of it because it doesn't make sense. And I'm learning now that he'll say yes when he really means no."

"Do you mean it doesn't make logical sense, or you just don't understand the words? Are they blurred together?"

"I try to tease it out and go along with whatever he says."

Trying to decipher Jim's thoughts can be stressful not only for Terri but also for Jim. Despite Jim being unaware of most of his actions, Terri does her best to keep Jim from getting frustrated. That is the case with many who have dementia. They are aware and angry when their words are not forming the proper way. To keep Jim's mind at ease, she prefers to have him focus on the aspects of life that always brought him peace. Terri finds that when she can connect serene moments for Jim, it's as if the disease subsides for a small moment.

"Does Jim have a special area that you consider his zen-zone? One care partner said they loved walking their dog on a nearby trail. Anything like that for Jim?"

Terri smiled as she thought of the two of them together. "Outside and with nature. When we were in Iceland, he was like, 'Oh my gosh, look at this, look at that. Look how beautiful that is.' When the leaves were turning, and we'd be driving, he would always say, 'Oh, look at that!'"

I pointed out that Jim and I have similar "happy places" in our love for fall. The leaves bring new light to Maryland and the air has the perfect level of crispness. Before I could sit down with Terri, I was with Jim on a long car ride to visit Mike, and I wish I had known then what I know about Jim now. Jim was quiet unless spoken to during our ride. I caught him in my rear view mirror staring out the window. Hoping he wasn't uncomfortable, I would pepper him with questions to keep him involved. He'd respond happily and clearly with one or two-word answers, then return to the window.

Thinking back to Jim that day reminded me of a story Mike told me about the first time he met Jim at a support group meeting. That night the group was set to gather at the house of a support group leader, Kathy, and her husband, Dave, who was diagnosed with another kind of young-onset dementia. Mike was eager to meet others like him but was extremely anxious about whether he would fit in with the other members. Then, Mike saw Jim.

"I must have driven past Kathy's house, then back to the hotel where I was staying, four times. Back and forth, back and forth, too afraid to go inside. I was so nervous!" Mike recalled with a familiar sense of nerves. "Finally, I knocked on the door, and when I entered the house, the first person I saw was Jim. He was like a lighthouse for me. He looked at me with a big smile and held his arms out. Once I saw him, I knew everything would be okay."

"Why do you call Jim a lighthouse, Mike?"

"That's what he was—what he is—like a lighthouse. Jim was this big, bright, shining image of hope, navigating me through rocky waters that night. If Jim wasn't there I don't know if I would have come back to the group again."

During my car ride with Jim, the leaves had already turned into a bouquet of burnt sienna, gold, russet, and crimson. A light morning rain gave way to a soft autumn sun that made everything glow from its damp reflection. Little did I know then that Jim wasn't being quiet out of worry but rather allowing the leaves to ease his mind. Terri told me after our trip to see Mike that Jim couldn't stop talking about how much he enjoyed the time with us. I was thrilled that the day gave Terri some optimism for Jim's health.

"Terri, this book is about Optimistics, but it goes further than just three buddies supporting one another. I know they each have their view of optimism, but how do *you* stay optimistic?"

Terri closed her eyes, then opened them, temporarily drying her tears.

"For me, I think I just take it day by day," she said, shrugging her shoulders. She smiled mid-thought and explained, "About two weeks ago, when all the kids were over, he caught me off guard."

"What do you mean?"

"Jim says to me, 'I like this,' and I said, 'What do you like, honey?' And he goes, 'When we're all together.'"

I could tell that was an emotional image for Terri. Hearing Jim say, "When we're all together," was something Terri knew would not be the same in a year. The topic of togetherness was a constant theme throughout this book, described as a critical element for the entire family's well-being. That conversation is all the proof needed to show that despite the little Jim does communicate or understand, the man they all knew for so long is still very much in there. He's changed but something in his heart reminded Jim that being with his family is what he loves more than anything.

When I told the Hursey family about finding a publisher for this book, Meaghan was the first person to email me back. She wrote, "I'm sitting in my car between patients—patients I treat with dementia—and I am in tears. This is amazing. To say I am excited for the future is an understatement."

I cried as well when I read her email.

I replied, "That means so much to me. This book has evolved into something I never would've imagined. It's incredible to have the support from everyone."

When Terri described Jim's love for nature, I couldn't help but think of him not being able to appreciate his comfort zone much longer. I will never be able to look at the changing of the leaves without thinking of Jim and I take that as a gift.

I hope that this upcoming autumn he will still be able to appreciate the colors in front of him.

I have an image of Jim in my mind, twirling the stem of a leaf with his fingers as the colors ricochet off his wide smile, with Terri holding his other hand tightly.

There is beauty in that image and I'll never let it go, no matter what changes come my way.

CHAPTER FOUR

Dennis

TIME IS IMPORTANT

"Dennis is like the Godfather of the group," Mike told me. Then he quickly added, "Well, between the Godfather and Mel Brooks."

There is something familiar about Dennis when you meet him. When someone talks about him, they usually do so by holding their hand over their chest saying, "Isn't Dennis just the sweetest?"

The first time I met Dennis in person, he skipped right past the handshake and hugged me like we were family. He felt like family right away. He also reminds me of my father, which plays a role in my connection to Dennis. He and my father have the same complexion and grew up in the same Jewish community. Each has a soft sensibility; they both wear thin metal glasses and have ear-to-ear smiles. Dennis has become known for his raspy tone as if he lost his voice the night before.

Like many people with Young-Onset Dementia (YOD), who had the decision to either live in the light or stay cornered in the darkness of their disease, Dennis chose the former. It wasn't overnight, yet his positivity has fueled the connections he formed through the Optimistics from their first meeting. As a Founding Father, Dennis's responsibility for the group is deeper than attending meetings, talking on the phone to others in his position, and being a brother to Jim and Mike. The continued growth of the Optimistics is Dennis's calling, and rightfully so since he spent his entire life helping people when they needed support the most.

"After we had been together for a short period, we wanted to push away this disease and fight it by coming up with things to be optimistic about. So, it was just natural to go out and become The Optimistics," Dennis said in an earlier conversation.

At sixty-eight, Dennis is the oldest in the group and the oldest Optimistic I've met thus far. Dennis knows about his age concerning his disease and speaks about his age as a matter of time he has left, not milestone numbers in years. Ironically, admiring time is something that has been a hobby of Dennis for decades. He has a large assortment of vintage watches at his house, kept in a box in the living room. Like any seasoned hobbyist, he couldn't wait to show me his elaborate collection. There were timepieces of different shapes, brands, styles, and colors. All had a story behind them, which I enjoyed hearing.

I think about Dennis's watches every time someone in the Optimistics discusses the concept of time. When he told me in an email that **time is important**, I knew it wasn't simply in passing. It's his reality. Being the elder statesman of the Optimistics also comes with the acknowledgment that statistically, his health is likely the first to feel the full brunt of dementia's force. Despite time ticking away quicker for Dennis than others, he does a fantastic job of ignoring Father Time.

For the Optimistics, Dennis has been anointed as their figurehead. When I first saw Dennis at the Alzheimer's Walk, he was the designated spokesman and commanded the crowd with his genuine outlook of optimism. Months before the Walk, their story caught the attention of a local Baltimore radio station. When all three of them were interviewed, Dennis led the charge. He did so not because he asked for it but because it's a part of his comforting demeanor that people are drawn to—like I was and still am today. Everyone, from his childhood to his coworkers, looked at Dennis as someone to rely on; in the medical field, it's a characteristic that comes naturally to him.

When I learned Dennis lived around the corner from me, I tried to visit often but also didn't want to intrude. I worked around their schedule to respect their routine. One of the many lessons I learned early on was the importance of working in a routine. "Similar to sleep training a baby," one person told me. I could relate to that analogy, having taken a drill sergeant-strict approach to sleep schedules for my two kids, or else all hell breaks loose.

I always enjoy spending time with Dennis and Judi because they feel at home or, better yet, remind me of family. Maybe it's our similar backgrounds or the inner workings of Jewish Smalltimore (as we Baltimoreans call the "small world" aspect of our busy city), but I feel like I've known Dennis and Judi forever. An early visit to their house allowed me a closer look into how Dennis lives today and what life was like before the diagnosis. I also learned quickly that Judi likes to cook, and I will leave with leftovers.

"Here, have a seat," Judi said, pointing to the kitchen island. "Do you like quiche? I'm making a quiche," she said, opening the oven.

"She makes a great quiche," Dennis said.

"Sure, I'd love some."

Judi smiled. "Good, because it's too big for just us. You'll take leftovers."

I guess I'm taking leftovers.

"How about some coffee? I can make some coffee," Dennis said.

"Coffee and quiche—I'm game."

I watched Dennis work the coffee maker on my behalf, with his hands slightly shaking as he placed the tiny cup into the machine.

"How are the kids? How's the family?" Dennis asked me as the machine revved to life.

"Good. We're all good, thanks."

I met Dennis midway to grab my coffee mug from him. "Tell them I said hi, please, will you?"

"Of course." I sipped my coffee and turned toward the oven, saying, "It's going to go well with my five slices of quiche, Judi.

*   *   *   *   *

The official diagnosis hit the medical professional in Dennis the hardest. Internally, Dennis knew something wasn't right. It's another smack of reality having a doctor sit across from you and lay the facts out on paper. As with every Optimistic I spoke to, they know they will have to forfeit certain aspects of their lives after diagnosis. Without fail, every interview I did for this book involved the topics of independence, being a provider, and having a career, which are the three main losses people with dementia feel the most. For Dennis, having lasted much longer than other Optimistics as a working professional, being sidelined before he had planned to retire was disheartening. As Dennis told me multiple times, medicine had been his passion since childhood.

When Dennis was nine, his parents bought him a toy doctor's bag with pretend medical instruments. That simple gift and practice of making pretend got Dennis hooked on being a doctor. Growing out of children's toys and into the serious world of medicine, Dennis spent decades as a Physician's Assistant, where he developed a bedside manner that made him a favorite amongst his patients. Since the beginning of his career, Dennis has been a success. Classmates and teachers admired him and later on, he became a go-to partner for every doctor he encountered. His approachable demeanor made it appear that Dennis could handle situations that would cause others at his level to fold under pressure. Alzheimer's began to slowly pick at Dennis's work-life balance, affecting his ability to operate his responsibilities in the office. For the first time, Dennis felt an unfamiliar stress that would eventually sideline him for good.

As a Physician's Assistant, part of Dennis's job included he complete a monotonous amount of paperwork that, as someone with tenure in the field, is secondhand and routine. At first, Dennis was behind on a few items until a few became many and alarmed others in the office. When his boss asked him about the paperwork lacking, Dennis quickly brushed off any concerns as a minor mishap and nothing major. He also promptly rectified concerns once they were brought to his attention. Dennis's reputation earned a level of respect that allowed him to fall behind without setting off too many alarms. However, even the best are being watched when it affects the whole practice.

Even though Dennis didn't want to admit the concerns to himself, he had to step down at sixty-eight, with only two years left before official retirement. For Dennis, who had always seen himself as a healer, having the tables turned to him needing care made for an uneasy transition. Although Dennis had to stop earlier than anticipated, he was able to work much longer than most people diagnosed with dementia, which for Dennis fell during the years defined for Young-Onset Dementia.

I asked Dennis about the initial days when he was forced into retirement, and in typical Dennis fashion, he remained optimistic.

"What else was I going to do?" he said, holding his hands out. "It wasn't their fault, and it wasn't my fault either."

As every Optimistic and care partner in this book will tell you, dementia is not something anyone should feel any sense of blame for. It's as random as rain and the remaining days are spent preparing for the unpredictable elements. Studies have shown that socialization, a healthy diet, exercise, and mentally stimulating challenges are positive ways to fight the possible effects of dementia. However, nothing is foolproof. When someone gets the diagnosis, they don't have the luxury to offer a rebuttal to the case, even though everyone tries.

—I can still do things on my own.

—A few more months of work and see if it gets better.

—Even if I stop working full-time, I can still work part-time.

—Even if I can't drive long distances, I can still drive to the store.

Unfortunately, the deep line of this disease is only drawn once, and there is no going back. The braver individuals know they have to move forward. Dennis was very honest about the end of his career, having made peace with the understanding that his body couldn't withstand his professional responsibilities any longer.

"Before you retired, did you notice any signs?"

Dennis swayed his head back and forth, trying to recall those days in greater detail. "I felt burnt out for sure."

He acknowledged lacking in certain areas of office protocol, but dementia was never a factor with the patients, the doctors, or the office staff. They always had a remarkable relationship with Dennis.

"The reason I stopped when I did was because if everything you've done is good, *don't* try to make it better." Dennis emphasized the word "don't" as if preaching from his own experience. "Like Johnny Unitas," Dennis offered, " you gotta go out on top."

Granted, Hall of Fame athletes have their own baggage when they leave their careers, and Dennis viewed his success in a manner that could have only gone worse if he had stayed on. Putting his ego aside for his health, he knew staying on any longer could negatively impact his immaculate tenure and tarnish his relationships with the community. Judi said Dennis's profound reputation around town has made him well known.

"People stop us when they see him."

Dennis loves these stories.

Judi chuckled while telling me about a recent interaction regarding Dennis and his fans. "This lady at the gas station ran up to him and said, 'Dennis! Dennis! Dennis! I miss you so much! There's nobody like you!' All because she loved seeing him at the doctor's office. This happens now and then," Judi added.

"He's a celebrity!" I said.

"Like you guys did at the Walk," she added, referring to Geoff and his mother approaching Dennis at the Walk to End Alzheimer's.

"You're totally right. Geoff and his mom gasped in awe when you popped up on stage. See, they were starstruck too!"

Dennis smiled and shrugged his shoulders.

"Fame. It comes with the territory, Dennis," I joked.

"He had over a hundred and fifty yamakas from all the bar and bat mitzvahs he's been invited to over the years. We had them forever but finally, we had to get rid of them. It was too much! He always collects stuff."

After a refill of coffee, Judi and Dennis start to poke fun at his hoarding and how it runs in his family.

"My mother was the one that started it," Dennis said in his defense.

"Yeah, but not as many yamakas, I bet," I said.

"There are some things you can't throw away," Dennis began, nodding his head as if he knew I'd appreciate the sentimentality of it. "I have a letter Mike wrote me that I've saved."

"For sure! You can't get rid of that."

"Well, yeah, because we're going to be famous," he laughed, then winked at me.

Along with Mike's letter, Dennis still has yamakas from his daughter's wedding and his own. He and Judi are in the middle of planning for their upcoming anniversary by crossing off one of Dennis's bucket list items.

"Any big plans for the anniversary?"

They both lit up with excitement.

"We're going to Ireland," Judi said.

"That's incredible!"

"We have another couple who have been good to us. They're both in the medical field, so they know his condition. Dennis used to work with both of them." Dennis nodded along.

"We're trying to do as much as possible," Judi added.

"Bucket list things," Dennis said.

"I'm jealous. Ireland is on my bucket list too."

"Don't wait," Dennis said with a knowing grin.

Judi looked at Dennis and asked, "Jim is going somewhere as well, right?"

"Iceland," said Dennis.

"Another place I want to go!" I screamed.

Dennis smiled, "See, bucket list."

During the time of this particular interview, I didn't realize the importance and urgency of checking off items on a bucket list for a person with dementia. I later asked Deb about this, and she pointed out the importance of making time now for events that Deb can't wait for later. It wasn't just Dennis and Jim planning elaborate vacations either; several other Optimists in the group had already done several bucket list items or had plans for the immediate future. Immediate is the keyword, as I pointed out during a meeting a month later.

At the meeting where bucket list vacations were celebrated, I sat next to Evie and told her I couldn't wait to see all the photos from their trips. She leaned in and reiterated my conversation with Deb, "A lot of people know they can't wait too long to make *those* plans." Evie knows this topic all too well, having gone on similar trips with her late husband, Mark.

I felt like an idiot when I realized why they rush their bucket list items. Whereas most people look at bucket lists for post-retirement life, the Optimistics have to work on an entirely different clock. Individuals with dementia and their care partners don't have the luxury of saying, "We'll do that next year."

Making sure they do their best to stay active while looking towards the future, Dennis and Judi have been fortunate to have friends around them. Not only do they have a good social circle stretching from childhood and college, but Dennis and Judi also have two incredible daughters who refuse to see their parents go down this road alone.

*   *   *   *   *

Lindsay

Lindsay was the first child of an Optimistic I connected with after I reached out to Judi. Judi sent my initial message to her daughters, and Lindsay held the velvet rope to Dennis. She was guarded initially since I was a stranger. Despite doing some Jewish Geography in the Baltimore area, linking myself to the Myers family on multiple levels, I still needed a direct connection to the family. More importantly, I hadn't earned the right to discuss the intimacies of Dennis's dementia.

Lindsay and I played email tag for several months and finally connected over a year ago. Admittedly, I was nervous about our interview, but that quickly became compassionate understanding. I saw her as a protector for her father, which I told her was a perfectly fine reason for her doubts. Within a few minutes, though, we both relaxed. I knew my role as a storyteller, and she believed in my mission for this book.

I learned quickly that Lindsay has a very analytical approach to Dennis's disease.

—*What needs to be done this week? What can each person in the family do?*

—*What is the immediate concern as of today?*

She's centered, grounded, and empathetic, yet doesn't have time for objections for the sake of making noise. She's the first one to let Judi know if she's being too dramatic or to make sure Dennis listens to Judi. Even though Lindsay and her family live in New York, the road home is not so far that she can't pick up and leave for her father when she has to. Distance hasn't stopped Lindsay's commitment to her father. She keeps an eye on Dennis, even from afar.

We spoke for over an hour and it was an eye-opening experience in life as the child of a YOD parent. She talked a lot about who Dennis was as a father growing up and accepting who he is today. She recognizes that things have changed, and they'll only distort into different knots the Myers family can't untie. Of all the things she sees differently in Dennis, it's his confidence that has been most impacted by dementia. After all, it was her father who could fix people's problems—including hers—yet now she's making sure his pains are minimized.

"I look at treating him like an individual versus just as my dad. Similar to how you see your kids as they go from infants to becoming their own person. I try to look at him now as an individual so I can better listen and support him based on what he truly needs and not necessarily what I'd expect or want or become accustomed to as his child."

Role reversal for parents with dementia and their children is another theme throughout an Optimistics' story and there is no correct way to approach it. Since every relationship is different, it's best to hear how others have adjusted their lives to make dementia more manageable and not to judge anyone for how long it took them to evolve. Who can be expected to wrap their brain around caring for a parent with dementia when you're still trying to figure out your own life? You can't critique a situation if you've never been in their position.

Lindsay said that people can't handle the pressure of a care partner role at first, and that's entirely fair, but what happens next is the difference between stepping up or sitting back as an observer. Lindsay had her challenges initially, as did her sister; however, the Myers women are not ones to watch from the sidelines.

"I try to focus on what we have with him now. I make now the focus and try to stay present versus focusing on anticipating what's to come."

Lindsay and I have met more than once since I entered their lives. In our first interview, she spoke about how hard it is to be around Dennis knowing he changes each day. When we met in person months later during one of her visits to Dennis and Judi's home, I could see the connection Lindsay has to her father on her face. We made small talk around the kitchen table, where Lindsay talked about Dennis being a caring father growing up.

"He's always been my greatest emotional support and one of the few people I feel like I can truly be myself around. We talked daily, and I never had to temper, sensor, or titrate myself around him."

Remaining authentic to yourself and your relationship with a person with dementia has become a separate battle, aside from the physical effects of dementia. The emotional toll it takes on someone like Lindsay, who lives five hours away and cares for her own children, grows daily. There is no quick fix to losing time with Dennis, even if their distance was closer. She remains hopeful that her time with him remains as positive as it can.

"How do you—or don't you—stay optimistic when it comes to seeing your dad live with dementia?"

"I cry when I need to," she said. "And try to create space for the tangle of emotions that come with this. I focus on our newer moments of connection to help fill some of the pits of what I've felt I've lost along the way. Ultimately, I'm trying to frame my focus on what I've got versus what I've lost."

Losing anything and everything to dementia comes in unpredictable as well as erratic waves. Everyone is helpless to its timing. You can only sit on the shoreline waiting to see how the tide settles, what was taken in the wake, and what you can do now to rescue the remaining pieces. The most challenging part for Lindsay is realizing what she'll miss most about him as things worsen is their pure connection.

"Along the way, to prepare for what is to come, I think I've worked to rely less on this part of our relationship—but it's honestly one of the things I miss the most. That and just the ease of talking."

*   *   *   *   *

Megan

The only things I knew about Megan before meeting her were that she was three years older than Lindsay and had the Hebrew school nickname "Megan the Pagan." Dennis and Judi said she received her contrarian moniker because she constantly challenged the rabbi about who God's parents were.

Megan rolled her eyes at her nickname. "I'm not really a pagan!" she said. "I just had questions. That's all."

Right off the bat, I liked Megan the Pagan. Like Lindsay, she's honest and direct, but whereas Lindsay seems to speak from the heart, Megan shoots from the hip. Like a comedian with blunt tones and casualness, Megan calls it like it is. Be it her professional or personal life, she doesn't have time for lazy people or those who get in the way. I could see early on that Dennis and Judi raised two empathetic and compassionate women. When it comes to Dennis's care, they will do whatever they need to for their father, each with a different approach.

When we met at a support group meeting, we didn't have a chance to discuss Dennis on a more personal level, so Megan and I made plans to meet at a quaint coffee shop by her house in Old Town Ellicott City, Maryland. Ellicott City can be described "as a dot on a dot on a map," with all the charm of small-town Americana sprinkled with some urban hipster. After grabbing our coffee and finding a small table, I told Megan to share whatever she wanted. This is her story, and I am only here to listen. The first thing she told me started the interview off in a rather unique manner.

Before my first sip of coffee, Megan holds her hands on the table to clarify her stance. "Listen, I am not a positive person."

She waited for my response as if her pessimism was a deal breaker. It wasn't. I laughed, not because her honesty was humorous, but because I'd heard the same statement from other care partners. I told them the same thing I told Megan, I'm not exactly Mr. Optimistic, which was another reason I wanted to write this book. It was my negativity that attracted me to Dennis and the other Optimistics in hopes they could guide me to better realize my anxiety in light of what I have in front of me. Making sense of optimism when the world seems to pin you down with financial worries, and concerns about your children, spouse, career, or personal growth can feel incredibly smothering even to a perfectly healthy person. As I explained to Megan, what happens when you take all of those same pressures and now pile on impending death decades before your time should come? With new health concerns added to your old worries, how can anyone stay calm in that storm?

We bonded over our mutual claims of pessimism and agreed that optimism is anything but natural or easy.

"Then I met the Optimistics," I told her.

Even as I write this journey, I'm still trying to place personal stresses into perspective against what the Optimistics face. With the Optimistics, finding optimism while living with dementia is the sole task. Keeping an overall enthusiastic mindset on all things about life is not necessarily a key factor, but for Optimistics, it has to be the best model to follow.

"Look, Lindsay may be optimistic, but I'm not," Megan added. "Lindsay is more like Dennis—tender, emotional, and will break down when thinking about Dad."

"And what are you?" I asked.

"I'm not like that—I'm a Judi."

We laughed together because I knew what she meant. Judi is incredibly sincere and warm, but in her role with Dennis, she has to be on the go. Judi is a fixer, a mover, and, as Megan agreed, a fighter.

We reflected on the fact that Judi is also the daughter of two Holocaust survivors, both of whom passed away before they had a chance to enjoy the full perks of parenthood, let alone being a grandparent. As a result, Judi had to make her way in handling struggles, and Megan credits Judi with accepting Dennis's diagnosis, as well as the future, as being better than anyone could expect.

"Were you surprised about the diagnosis?"

"Not really," she said half-jokingly. "He was at retirement age anyway, and this was way before the diagnosis. But no. I mean, with him getting diagnosed, I wasn't surprised. I knew it had to be something."

All of the Myers women agreed the signs were there, but Dennis's mind needed to speak up. We also discussed whether they wished they had found this out years before. Anyone would want to know sooner. Having discovered his illness later in life, the remaining time with Dennis is now down to a day-by-day schedule, as dementia's timetable answers to no one.

"What about the internal clock that dementia puts on people? The harsh reality is there is no cure. Does that change your thinking?"

"Not really. I mean, even though I'm practical," she said with a smile. "And I'm good at complaining about things in my life that are really, in the grand scheme of things, not that big of a deal. It's like we have all the more reason to spend time with him. Also, all the more reason not to get as frustrated with him. It makes me want to be around him even more."

I pointed out that's ironically a very optimistic viewpoint. Megan rolled her eyes, refusing to accept defeat. She knows that even with the most laid-back approach to accepting this diagnosis, there will come a time when being around Dennis will be difficult.

"When he forgets who I am…" she paused for the first time, "that'll be really hard."

Then, quickly after that, Megan bursts into the positive.

"He's had a great life! He's seen us get married, he's seen us have kids. The other people haven't. Some have teenagers!"

She's right about Dennis's age concerning his condition, which has allowed him to live the grandparent experience most Optimistics will never have, even if they are still alive. When we talked about family, though, she told me Dennis worries about his future as a figurehead in the family.

"He sometimes feels like he's disappearing into the background."

Megan said Dennis feels this way because they usually call Judi's cell phone when she and Lindsay call home.

"I'm like, okay, Dad, well, I'll start calling you instead of Mom. I hear him in the background saying 'Hi,' so I want to make sure he doesn't feel like he's fading into the background."

I poked around for more reasons Dennis felt like he was fading into his family's background. Megan told me a story about their recent Thanksgiving dinner. The extended Myers family is known to host a large Thanksgiving every year, with four generations gathered together at a local country club to celebrate the holiday as one. This past Thanksgiving, Megan said, was different for Dennis.

"People would come up to me and say, 'Hey, Mego, how's Dad doing? Is everything okay?' I'm like, 'Yeah, look at him! He's good.' It's as if they can't ask themselves," Megan added sarcastically.

Dennis heard the whispers that day, regardless of how discrete people tried. The silence that surrounds dementia is something only those living with it can ever fully comprehend. Regardless of age, everyone in this book said people around them were too afraid to mention their diagnosis. As a result, dementia continues to have a negative connotation about someone, as if life must stop with the diagnosis, allowing others to avoid them altogether. So, they fade. And as Dennis said, he fears becoming transparent to those around him and is cognizant of watching it happen.

How can you stay optimistic with that level of emotion?

As the Optimistics tell me repeatedly, "You have to."

Even though Megan's initial wall was held up by a persona of realistic expectations towards dementia rather than positivity, not everyone in an Optimistics' life can remain blocked from hope. As many people mentioned to me, there is a darkness that comes with this disease, and the fear of allowing that to take over is the only push you need to go forward. Megan's personality likes to be challenged, and I wanted to revisit the topic of staying optimistic when she thinks about Dennis.

She shrugged her shoulders. "It's easy for me to stay optimistic with Dennis because he's my dad. As a parent, I respect him a thousand times more than I ever did. I want to take care of him because he took care of me. That, and *he's* optimistic! He's always smiling, so it's kind of infectious. It's hard not to be positive around him."

*   *   *   *   *

Although he no longer has an office to practice, the caring professional in Dennis has not stopped him from helping others daily. Whether through a text, a phone call, or in person, Dennis checks in on his fellow Optimistics. He asks how their family is doing, and how they're holding up, and he always tries to keep others smiling. Even though he's doling out the optimism, Dennis also remembers his self-check-up. He knows what it's like to have Father Time pull you into the shadows and make you less visible to those around you. To fight back against dementia's clock, Dennis smiles through the pain so he can gain more time to be with his family.

This year, Dennis and Judi will celebrate their 45th wedding anniversary, surrounded by their loved ones, with the bright spotlight shining directly onto them—and far away from the darkness.

CHAPTER FIVE

Mike

OUR GENERAL WASHINGTON

"How do you spell LIFE? T.I.M.E." Mike shook his head slowly, knowing that time was his key to living despite a catalog of illnesses that left him at death's doorstep on more than one occasion.

To say Mike is an anomaly compared to the other Optimistics is an understatement. He has managed to defy many of the serious setbacks of Young-Onset Dementia (so far), allowing him to live an incredibly independent life. It's one thing to be self-sufficient while dealing with dementia, which in itself is a mild victory, and another to do so when you take into account Mike's lack of support. He has no care partner or children. His closest family members are his mother and sister, who live over 230 miles away from him in New Jersey. Mike still manages his finances, doctor's appointments, and social calendar. To further stress how incredible Mike is, any of those qualities would be an epic achievement for someone with YOD.

Once you meet Mike, you won't be surprised by his accomplishments. Mike is the most poetic, openly emotional Optimistic, with very poignant philosophies of how YOD has affected his life. One minute he's talking about a movie or TV show, then George Washington and Benjamin Franklin. Next, he'll open up into an eloquent monologue about how the Optimistics have helped him focus on the happier sides of life. For someone who calls himself an introvert, Mike doesn't hold back when it comes to expressing what he's feeling. One time, he told me, "Alzheimer's robs your dignity, kills your spirit, and kills you from the inside out."

No other Optimistic can generate the imagery of how YOD has changed their lives like Mike continues to do. Even though he will say that the diagnosis can crush your will, his natural ability to speak about dementia landed him as the Speaker of the Optimistics. Dennis may be the Godfather, but Mike knows how to gather the troops. His poise in front of people brought him to the doors of the Health & Human Services building in Washington, D.C. to speak about the need for better assistance with lifesaving dementia medication. On a March evening last year, organized by the support group, Mike stood with a megaphone to share his story. Although he'll admit he was incredibly nervous, you could never tell.

"I had a piece of paper with my notes, but I didn't even use it. I just spoke from my heart," he said, as if the whole day was an out-of-body experience.

Hearing Mike talk about how his heart has guided his self-belief is reassuring, considering he has no immediate sounding board at home. Mike's story takes center stage when he's around the support group and other Optimistics. I've seen that version of him over the past year amplified when he has a smaller audience who knows what he's going through personally. One night after a meeting, I took Mike and Dennis to a cozy roadside coffee shop called the John Brown Coffee to talk about the Optimistics. The three of us sat at a small table in the back for more privacy.

Mike tells people he's an introvert, but once he opens up, the real Mike emerges, as it did with his trek to D.C. We looked at some pictures from that day on his phone, and he remembers that day well. He said his goal was to connect with the politicians and let them see that the YOD community is strong but needs help. Mike also wanted them, and everyone else, to understand that dementia is a family disease. Most of us has a connection to it through even the slightest relationship in their lives.

"When I asked that young staffer, 'What's your relationship with Alzheimer's?' She looked at me and said nothing." Mike held his hands open, still scared and dumbfounded by her absence of a quality response.

Mike pointed his finger at the table like a podium on a stage. "So right there, that tells me, how are *you* going to approach this? This way, that way? How do you approach a young kid who knows nothing about dementia? You've got to get that message to someone like her," he said, referring to the young staffer. "Because she's the conduit between us and that Congressperson who can do something about it. That way, the changes aren't going to get lost."

While Mike can speak with a refined intensity about his illness for hours, he is a jokester first and foremost. He doesn't mind telling a joke, throwing around a curse word here and there, and laughing at himself. He enjoys giving people nicknames, usually related to something from pop culture. Mike dubbed one of the other Optimistics in the support group "Ted Lasso " because they always have witty one-liners, just like Ted's character. Mike nicknamed me "Secret Squirrel" because he said my gold aviator sunglasses and dark jacket made me look like a Secret Service agent. I told Mike I'd be a lousy spy, but he said I just had to look the part. I didn't bother to ask about the squirrel bit. Whether through work or with friends, he is genuine to the bone, and everyone who has met him will say the same thing.

Mike lives in Solomons Island, Maryland, a charming, Hallmark Channel-esque gem on the southern point of the Chesapeake Bay. Like many small beach towns, Solomons Island is primarily a summer destination, and even then, it's more of a pass-through visit compared to the more popular oceanfront beaches along the Maryland and Delaware coasts. Everyone on the island knows each other through work, seeing one another at a bay side restaurant, or strolling along the narrow boardwalk downtown.

Mike moved there decades ago to work as an aviation engineer, servicing military and commercial helicopters. He instantly fell in love with island life. Work and the small town culture allowed him to value an independent life with two main passions: his faith and career. As the latter would be taken away by YOD, the former would guide him in a comfortable direction to find peace. It was also God who Mike turned to when his health began to decline. Right before the pandemic, Mike was walking his dog Jasper, when he started to feel dizzy. He took a few steps, then collapsed in the dirt. Mike was rushed to the hospital where he was told he had suffered a heart attack. He was lucky they got to him in time, especially considering his medical history. A few years before his heart attack, Mike battled prostate cancer.

Shortly after Mike returned home from heart surgery, he said he started to notice memory loss here and there. "Nothing major," he thought at first, and Mike, being Mike, continued to go about his life. Gradually, his memory loss became more regular until finally, Mike couldn't ignore the signs.

"Everything changed for me practically overnight."

His eyelids flickered, trying to hold back tears. "I started seeing some of the stuff that I was missing, like with the job, working on helicopters. I had to admit that I really couldn't do it anymore."

"Was there a certain moment that made you finally admit it to yourself?"

"Yeah. One day, I just walked right by my helicopter and didn't even know it was there."

Mike still can't get over how obvious of a sign that event was to him. He stretched his long arms out to express the magnitude of the helicopter for me and Dennis. "When you walk by a helicopter that's the size of this coffee shop," he said, looking around. "I didn't know where I was at. How did I do that?"

Like every person I talked to, Mike did his best to ignore the obvious signs of dementia. He soldiered on, yet that battle became futile. One day he was walking around his neighborhood and couldn't remember how to get home. Another time, he was out running an errand and when he got back into his car, he realized he didn't know where he was. Mike called an old military friend who pinged his location through his phone and then guided him home. Situations such as those kept popping up to the point where Mike had to realize it was time to see a professional.

He still gasps about his first appointment with a doctor over his shock about the results. "I couldn't believe it! I mean, what else could be wrong with me? Cancer, heart attack, and now Alzheimer's?"

Cancer, heart attack, and YOD—all before the age of sixty.

In Mike's mind, he didn't think it was fair and he's right, it's not. Mike's one, two, and three punches of medical illnesses were about to worsen. While at the doctor they thought he may have Lewy Body Dementia. On top of memory loss this can also cause tremendous physical limitations, similar to Parkinson's disease. This includes tremors, moving slowly, and rigidity in muscles. However, Lewy Body Dementia often starts with visual hallucinations and dementia prior to Parkinson's like symptoms beginning. Not only did the fear of this throw Mike into hysterics, but the scarier part was his father died of congestive heart failure and dementia. Mike felt his time was ending, just as his father's did.

"When they gave me a CT scan, the doctor said that Alzheimer's was eating away at my brain." Mike's mouth hung open as if the muscles were cut from his face. His eyes grew wide at remembering how unexpected his entire diagnosis was to embrace.

I put my hand on Mike's arm. "I can only imagine what it was like being told you have the same diagnosis as your father."

"To watch my dad go through that—it just hurt. Now, I have a front-row seat to Alzheimer's. This disease plays for keeps and doesn't give back," he said in a reflective tone.

It was later shown that Mike did not have Lewy Body Dementia, but the concept still affects his psyche today. When he talks about his late father, Mike mentions his mother in the same breath. Now in her mid-eighties, he constantly worries about her. He'll talk about the importance of her care rather than his own and will visit her in New Jersey as much as he can. One thing he points out about his mother is how destroyed she was by his father's death and it's her words after his passing that has created a unique dynamic to Mike's openness about his condition.

"My mom doesn't know about my dementia, and I will not tell her. No way. I can't do that to her," he said admittedly. "When my dad died, she said she can't handle any more bad news. If anyone has bad news, she doesn't want to hear about it. So, I'm not going to tell her."

Although Mike keeps his diagnosis from his mother, his sister is aware of everything. She helps him when she can, and together they are working to support their mother and Mike. Between the support group, his fellow Optimistics, and his sister, Mike knows he has a lot of support.

Yet, distance has strained his ability to stay connected with everyone. As a result, he courageously discusses his battles with depression due to that isolation. Deb, Evie, and I have talked about finding him a home in Baltimore so he's closer to the medical assistance he needs as well as the emotional support required for his mental health. Mike is very open to the idea. As I write this, we're working on finding the best avenues to improve his living conditions. He may live independently, but everyone in the support group empathizes with him regarding the isolation he lives with daily.

Isolation is a dangerous area for care partners and individuals with dementia. Everyone I met brought up the topic of loneliness when discussing their lives, and I can't help but picture what life is like for them. In every situation, the feeling or reality of isolation comes to mind for both sides. Even if they still live together, the wall that YOD creates between the person with dementia and their care partner will forever be a transparent facade. They can see the person they always knew, but that person has changed and will likely worsen. Whereas someone with dementia may be unable to comprehend the amount of pain the care partner is enduring, care partners themselves can't escape the mental solitude felt on their side of that wall.

For the Optimistics, their jobs are gone due to forced retirement, their independence has been revoked, and they are at the mercy of someone telling them what to do and where to go. Mike is more aware of his condition than the other Optimistics and there is a sense of torture in that notion. While others have faced the way dementia has relinquished their autonomy, Mike waits for his time when the luxury of his independence is stolen from underneath him. With that in mind, I'm in awe of how he embraces every day with the positivity that has become his calling card. Yet, there are times when I see the sadness in how Mike views his routine now compared to what it was pre-diagnosis. I find he tends to correlate his post-diagnosis regime as being the result of losing everything he enjoyed about life prior.

"I don't like being out of work. I love working. I love doing stuff. I try to do as much as possible to keep my mind active."

I turned back to the positive and focused on how Mike lives each day since he is the embodiment of an Optimistic. I told him how lucky he was to have friends like Dennis, Jim, and the Optimistics group, which wasn't lost on him. He is the first to talk about how the Optimistics saved his life and gave him a new purpose. The bond he's created through the group is better than any prescription.

"We talk about the demands of going through this ordeal but try to offset it by talking about topics that are fun—uplifting—as well as some of the things that are scary about the disease."

"It has to make you feel so good about how the group has grown since you started, right?"

"Oh, yeah! We talked about that today on our group phone call. The Optimistics are getting bigger now. We were on the radio!"

"Yeah, you started a trend," I said.

"It's funny, but all these people are joining the group. They're like, 'Well, we heard you guys on the radio,' and I couldn't believe it," Mike said laughing. "Like, oh, shit, look what's happened! It's like, what the hell do we do now?"

I patted him on the back. "You should be very proud, Mike."

"Hey, we're like the Beatles of dementia, man," he added.

"That could be your new tagline, The Optimistics: The Beatles of Dementia," I said, motioning my hands as if the words were in lights.

The idea of a tagline for the Optimistics led him to a story from a late friend whose life was cut short due to cancer. Before his passing, Mike said his friend taught him the value of finding humor daily while going through a medical battle.

"He passed away when he was like thirty-five or forty, and before that happened, we were kids amongst ourselves. Let's say we were going to park the car, and I'd say, 'You're not going to fit your car in that little amount of space,' and then he'd get it in on the first try. Then he would say he was just fucking lucky."

All three of us laughed at his silly story about an old friend and how incredible it was for his friend to consider himself lucky during his illness. However, as it goes with Mike, you never know what he will say next. Then, he hits Dennis and me with another gem. Mike held up his finger to tell us he had a great idea. "What about The Fucking Lucky Club for our tagline? We can get that on a t-shirt."

I truly believe he was only half joking.

"Well, that can be a problem, Mike," I told him, hoping not to burst his bubble.

"Yeah, I can see that. But hell yeah, I think that would be a good title for your book, Richie!"

"I'll write that down. Kind of like, *The Joy Luck Club*, but now we're the *Fucking Lucky Club*."

"Yeah, like that!" he said.

"I think you're doing more than enough with the name you have now, Mike—all of you. It just takes someone, or a group, to put themselves out there, to lead the charge," I said.

"I think so. The same people see all about the frailties of dementia, and I think that's what hits them hard. I remember my favorite story is about George Washington. I love this story."

Mike leaned back on his chair and crossed his thick arms over his barreled chest. "When was it? I think it was at the Newburgh Address. Washington had hired soldiers and mercenaries who worked in the Army, and they were coming up on their one-year commitment, and then they were done. They were losing battles, not getting paid, and things didn't look good."

Mike moved forward, putting his elbows on the table as if he were in the war himself, retelling it to a classroom of little kids.

"But Washington needed his men, so he came out, and he talked to the guys, and he said something like, 'I want to talk to everybody together,' and all his troops ran up. Then Washington removed his spectacles and said, 'I have grown not only gray, but almost blind in the service of my country.'"

Mike went on to tell us about how Washington took his troops from their lowest points to build their confidence to fight on. He added, "Then the soldiers decided not to go. They stayed with Washington and fought." Mike looked at me and Dennis for reassurance in the meaning of his story. Of the many lessons I've learned from Optimistics, one is never to interrupt a story, even if I don't quite understand the meaning behind its message. I asked Mike what made him think of Washington.

He said, "I feel like we're in the same time as them, right now. I feel like we're talking to the same people in our group, the same state, and we're going out again. It's like we need to tell the people in the group and others in the community,

'We need you, don't leave us. We need more of you to fight for us.'"

There it is. That's Mike.

"That's beautiful," Dennis said in his soft graveled voice.

I told Mike how much I appreciate his passion for Optimistics and being a champion for dementia. Mike told me that it's his job now. Things have changed, but he still can work for something greater than himself.

Like most with dementia, Mike didn't choose to leave work; he was forced to do so, not by his boss, his coworkers, or the company, but by the nature of the responsibility that comes with a YOD diagnosis. For years, Mike searched for a way to work just as hard as he always did and provide himself with the feeling of accomplishment that comes with a successful career. He knew his life would be forever altered when he could no longer call himself an engineer, but he also picked up a new title that may create a lasting legacy.

"My identity has changed, and there are lots of good things about me that I can take with me."

Like the soldiers who fought for Washington, who had to believe in a mission for the country's greater good, Mike sees what he's doing with the Optimistics as a similar journey in helping others.

"You're like General Washington," I told Mike. "You have to stand up for the cause."

"Thanks, Richie. So, if we," Mike said, pointing to me and Dennis as symbols of the Optimistics' movement, "don't want to go, then no one will listen. We have to do it."

Mike pointed to us again. "*You* have to do it!"

As of writing this chapter, Mike is still living an independent life on Solomons Island. He regularly attends church, is always available for his mother and sister, and shows no signs of giving up the good fight. His advocacy efforts have paid off as well. Mike's speech in D.C., arguing against disgustingly overpriced dementia medications, was successful enough to help lower costs and is now covered by Medicare.

We all salute you, Mike, our own General Washington.

CHAPTER SIX

Karla and Michael

THE GIRL FROM MANAUS

The first thing Michael will tell you about Karla is how talented an engineer she was for decades. As an ophthalmologist himself, with a flourishing career in his own right, Michael believes his work pales compared to what Karla has accomplished. That self-deprecating humor is a vital part of Michael's charm. He humorously knocks himself down several notches when he gets a chance to brag about Karla.

"Look, I'm not a dummy, but in medical school, you have to read, you have to learn things, and you have to know how to use it. That's not the same as saying, 'We're changing the pipe size to this diameter,'" Michael said, pinching his finger and thumb together. "What are the risks of an explosion if we're changing this chemical formula or something? It was her job to make that work. She was such a brilliant chemical engineer, so she's that smart. I couldn't do that."

I have heard Michael speak about Karla at YES group meetings and met her several times in the last year and a half. At the 2023 Walk To End Alzheimer's in Baltimore, I sat next to them during the opening ceremony. On stage was a fellow group member, Nancy. She was speaking about her sweet husband, Marty, who was living with a severe level of dementia, affecting his speech and comprehension. Before she went up, Nancy asked if I could sit close to the stage so she could have more support, which I was more than happy to do. As she spoke, her eyes watered despite her incredible confidence and poise while she told her story of Marty's battle in front of hundreds of strangers. Marty stood with his arm around her, admiring her strength.

Even then, Michael made time to use his sarcasm. For the Walks, people are given different colored plastic windmill flowers to show their support. Blue is for those who are currently experiencing Alzheimer's Dementia. Purple indicates if you've lost a loved one to the disease. Yellow is for the fantastic caregivers. Orange represents anyone who believes in a future without dementia. Michael moved his bag with a collection of windmills so I could sit next to him. "I got all of these. Which one do you want? I got purple, I got blue, I got orange, I got yellow, you name it. You want one—I'm your guy." Then he smiled and winked.

Michael leaned over to Karla. "You remember, Richie, Kar?" he said to Karla, or Kar as he called her.

Karla shined in the warm fall weather and smiled back at me.

"Of course she does," I said. "Hi, Karla!" I waved.

I knew she didn't remember me, but that wasn't the point.

Michael is usually the only male care partner at the support meetings. He always comes from work dressed in khakis, a button-down shirt loosened for comfort, and a tie dangling down his lean frame. During the sessions, Michael sits cross-legged talking fast with his hands, painting pictures for his words. Even when topics such as Karla's care become hard to handle, he still threw in a funny comment to lighten the mood. For most of my time at the support meetings, Karla was always with Michael until recently. The group became too hard for her, yet Michael still attends.

Even though I have spoken with him at every meeting, I never heard about his life with Karla. We set up a time to grab breakfast at a kosher bagel shop called Goldberg's, which has been a staple in Baltimore for decades. I learned early on that Michael and I have a lot in common. For starters, we agreed Goldberg's wears the crown when it comes to who's the king of bagels in Baltimore.

"Without a doubt, these are the best," Michael said, taking a bite of his bagel.

"I'm with you, 100%," I nodded. "Can you believe some people still buy bagels from grocery stores?"

Michael held up his hand. "Stop! It's a shame," he added with a smile.

When he smiles, it makes you want to smile.

Michael is a regular here and throughout our visit, he said hello to at least half a dozen people. He even joked about his love for carbs.

"You know Peter Sellers from *The Pink Panther*? Inspector Clouseau?"

"Yes, I'm familiar."

"What he did was wrong, but he said the words I live by."

"What's that?" I asked unsurely.

"His doctor told him, 'Peter, you've got to stop drinking, smoking, and womanizing, or you're going to die.' Well, that's not the right stuff to do, but his answer was, 'You've got to live before you die, or you'll die before you live.' So, if I want a bagel, I will have a bagel."

I almost spit out my coffee at Michael's analogy.

"I watch my sugar the best I can. I go to a personal trainer, but I'm having my dessert. You know, I don't want to kill myself off or anything," he added with his arms held out.

"I think you'll be okay with eating bagels, Michael."

Somehow, Michael can talk about death with a touch of humor.

"Were you and Karla eating better for her future health? I have heard from many care partners that eating healthier is a good way to lessen the impact of dementia."

"Eh, we tried," he said flippantly. "Did I ever see her get better? No. Did she continue to deteriorate? Yes, but I did try it."

Then Michael became rather giddy out of nowhere, "But I ended up with the coolest product ever." He snapped his fingers, trying to remember the name of the device. "Oh, come on," *snap-snap-snap*. "It looks like a toaster oven, and they send you food like raw chicken breast and vegetables like broccoli or potatoes."

Snap-Snap-Snap.

Then it hit him, "The Tovala Smart Oven!" He clapped his hands together.

When listening to Michael's delivery, I felt like I was having breakfast with Larry David or Steve Martin as he got on a run about a topic he enjoyed. "So that we would eat in rather than going out for Chinese and Mexican food and stuff every night," he continued.

"Like an air fryer?"

"This is better. And what you do is you put it in the little tin that they send you, and then they give you a recipe card, and the oven reads the QR code, and it'll go from bake to broil to air fry to steam. You name it, it's great!"

"It sounds cool, but I don't cook."

Michael leaned in, his eyes wide. "Well, look, if you decide to do it, put my name in because then you get an extra credit," he said, taking a bite of his bagel. I'll email you a link."

That's such a Larry David thing to say.

"Sounds like a deal," I said.

Since Michael was living alone, the excitement he felt from appliances that could make his life more manageable after a busy day was surely needed. However, before Karla's illness captured her body, I was curious if Karla ever brought some of her Brazilian heritage into the kitchen. Michael smiled as he remembered one of their first conversations, which was actually about cooking.

"When Karla and I first met, she said, 'Look, before we get married, you have to know this about me. I'm a chemical engineer. I know how to mix blue with yellow to make green, but I don't know how to cook.'"

We both erupted with laughter.

"And she was right!" he said. "And all I could cook were tacos and burritos."

"Well, there you go. You were made for each other."

Michael took another bite, then said, "Richie, she was really funny. Especially when she made fun of herself, you know? Everyone loved being around her."

"From what you said at the YES meetings, it seemed like she always got along with everyone."

"Oh yeah. She would have friends call up and say, 'I don't know what to do with this girl I'm dating.' Karla would say, 'Don't worry. Come over here, sit down, and talk to me.' She has a tremendous amount of insight into everything.

Then Michael paused for a moment. "Now, it's all gone," he said, shrugging his shoulders.

"Can you tell me how you guys first met?"

"Interestingly, I was going to see my family in Houston, Texas, to stay for a week or two. Karla was with her professor from Israel, where she was living and studying, for a conference," Michael began before being interrupted by an old friend walking by. "See ya, guys! Yup, I'll be here tomorrow," he shouted to them.

Michael faced back in my direction. "Anyway, if you know anything about Texas, it's so darn big that when you're done with your family - if they love you - they drive you back to the airport." I was sensing his Larry David tone coming around again. "But, if they're my family, they take you to the shuttle at Neiman Marcus and wait for three hours as it drives around and ends up at the airport… eventually."

I was losing it more and more with every one-liner Michael delivered.

I pictured Michael in his early twenties, waiting for the airport bus to appear, knowing it would be a while, and cursing his family for their "gratitude" as he kicked small pebbles along the curb. I didn't envision how that one bus ride would change his life forever.

"Then, on the bus, Karla ended up sitting next to me, but she didn't want to tell me anything about herself because she heard that people in the south were anti-semitic."

Like Michael, Karla is Jewish and was raised around a tight faith-based community called Manaus in a small Brazilian city in the Amazon. Growing up, her family was only one out of one hundred Jewish families in a city of a million. Even though she went to college in America, where she met people of all religions, she still encountered antisemitism, so her natural guard was still up around new people.

"But, little by little," Michael said, "she told me, 'I'm from Manaus.' Then she showed me a picture of her people in a canoe. She said, 'Here's my family, you know, Indians.'"

When Karla described the isolated area of her youth, Michael envisioned he life she described: one in a canoe in the middle of the Amazon jungle without the perks of technology or entertainment. After all, this was hardly something Michael was used to hearing from the girls he dated before.

Despite her tight-knit upbringing, her family's history of tremendous business success allowed Karla, her brother, and others in the family to pursue highly-skilled degrees in science, business, and medicine. From surgeons, doctors, engineers, and CEOs, Karla's lineage taught her to always chase after what your passions were, no matter how far away from home they may take you.

Michael and Karla talked the entire ride to the airport and seemingly hit it off. Michael realized the distance between their lives would likely mean he'd never see her again. Still, he gave it a shot.

"I was getting ready to leave the bus and told Karla, 'If you're ever back in the United States, give me a call.'"

"That was it? How long did it take to speak with her again?"

"A few months—not long," Michael said lightly as if it was a week. "One night, I got a phone call from a woman with a big accent."

I stopped taking notes, "I never caught onto Karla's accent when speaking to her at the support group meetings."

Michael smiled. "She speaks much softer and infrequently now, so you may not notice it. But it was a very thick accent for a while. Then, I get a call at three o'clock in the morning," Michael said, rolling his head around like, 'Who the heck is calling me at three o'clock in the morning?!'

Michael admitted he was not exactly thrilled to be woken up so early. Michael's interpretation of that call was as spot on as I imagined him reacting. He told the voice on the other line, "Ma'am, I have to work tomorrow. It's 3 a.m.!"

Then the voice on the other end said, "What's your name?"

Michael was so frustrated that he cut the caller off. "This is Michael Sandler. You have the wrong number."

Yet, before Michael could hang up, the voice on the other end said, "No. You're the one." Michael repeated it, "I'm the one."

He sat up in bed like Dracula popping out of a coffin when he realized the beautiful woman he had given his phone number to on the bus had followed up on his offer. "I was shocked!" he said.

Karla spoke in a delicate Portuguese accent. "You told me to call you when I'm going to be in Washington."

Michael could hardly make sense of the moment. "How do I have time to go to Washington?" But Karla remembered me saying, 'You said you would come if I returned to the States.' I just knew I had to go," he said.

He took a moment to praise Karla's intelligence again. "I went to D.C., and then she was accepted into the PhD program at Columbia University—Ivy League," he added, raising his eyebrows.

"That's impressive," I told him. "How was life in New York?"

Michael started to laugh with a mouthful of bagel and cream cheese. "She didn't complete her PhD there."

"Why?"

"She was allergic to pigeons, and in New York, there are pigeons everywhere," he said, throwing his hands forward and further expressing the humor of the situation.

I shook my head, feeling he was pulling my leg. "How was she allergic to pigeons?"

"Yup. She kept going to the hospital and the doctors would shoot her up; she would have trouble breathing, then would get a rash."

"I have never heard of anybody being allergic to pigeons, Michael."

He held his hands out and said, "Well, now you have."

During that time, Michael was living in Baltimore while Karla struggled through the pigeon-infested streets of Columbia University. They would swap visits. Eventually, the steroids Karla was taking for her allergies became too much, and she could no longer tolerate New York.

Karla called Michael one day and told him, "Either I come to live with you in Baltimore, or I'll move back to Israel." With her family living halfway across the country, Michael was the only thing keeping her in the States. So, Karla moved in with Michael. He worked in his practice, and she took a high-level job as a Chemical Engineer. Eventually, they were married and grew their family by two children: a son, Evan, and a daughter, Elana. Life was perfect for Michael and Karla, but he still can't believe it happened on a random bus ride in Texas.

"The odds of us meeting," Michael said, rolling his eyes, "it was unbelievable."

"See, you thought your family was being lazy by dropping you off at Neiman Marcus!" I said.

He laughed, "Good point."

Having been with Michael and Karla at meetings, I admired how he can keep up his sense of humor despite Karla's noticeable decline. He would sit next to her closely, repeat questions to her, and then add an answer for her with a smile as if it was Karla's doing. Their bond is infectious, as any true love should be, but as Karla's dementia progressed, Michael knew he had to find another alternative for her to receive the best care possible.

"She's at a living facility right by the house. I can visit whenever I want to or take her out."

"How old is she now?"

"Sixty-four."

"When was she diagnosed?

"Around four or five years ago," Michael said, with his hands over his chest. She's the sweetest and younger than most other residents there," he said lovingly. She sees people trying to get out of their chairs and runs to help them."

"She seems happy?"

"I don't know because if she sees somebody else, like one of our friends going over to say, 'Karla, how are you?' she'll go over and hug them. Karla will say, 'I love you, I miss you...' but I don't know. I mean, her condition is progressing."

Karla's symptoms began to show in her mid-fifties, with little things that made Michael concerned. Over time, it was clear that her memory was fading, even though her personality still seemed upbeat. As Michael said, many people tend to get violent or lash out, but Karla remains as soft as ever. With the kids grown and out of the house and Michael working in his practice, he hired caretakers to watch Karla while he was gone. At first, he thought it was precautionary, but it was clear to everyone that Karla's condition wasn't subsiding. It was speeding up.

Michael recalled some of the earlier signs of Karla's dementia. "I would get calls from neighbors who knew Karla saying, 'Michael, your wife is out here, and she doesn't know how to get home,' which was scary. I would ask them to please take her home because a caretaker will be there soon."

Michael was fortunate to have good support around him. "This disease brings out the bad in the person and the good in other people...and I'm not talking about the people that don't want to deal with it."

I reminded Michael how lucky he was to have such an optimistic team of people around him. After hearing stories from others in the support group, he felt that way as well. "I say this a lot, Michael, but dementia doesn't play favorites. It doesn't choose anyone, and neither does cancer. I mean, sure, if you smoke, your chances are increased. If you're an adventure seeker, Alpine off-the-grid skier, or skydiver, you may have some bad medical issues, but that's on you. You did that. Dementia just fires at random."

Michael took a sip. "Yeah, it's still…" His throat began to narrow. "See, I'm tearing up," he said, smiling. "It's quite an emotional thing."

"We can take a break if you want?" I offered.

"Please, you think I care about people seeing me cry," he laughed.

"I'm with you," I added. "It should be okay to get emotional in front of others. One of the biggest things that attracted me to the three Optimistics was that men finally talked about this stuff. Even for you, you're usually one of a few men at the meetings."

Michael wasn't always the sole husband at our support group meetings. He befriended a man named Frank who was a part of the group before my joining. Frank stopped coming to the support group after his wife passed away from Alzheimer's Dementia. Michael called Frank his "guru" because Frank always had the latest research on medications, dementia news, and treatment ideas. Frank joined Michael at a care partner-centered therapy treatment, and they bonded over various aspects of life. Care partners need that level of support, and Michael enjoyed his connection with Frank as a release from his situation. Even though Franks' wife was much farther along than anyone else, he always encouraged

Michael to remain positive. Sadly, Frank lost momentum as his wife entered her final stage of dementia.

After hearing about Frank, I told Michael I was happy he stayed with the group even though others had left. "More men come to the group. Lorinn's boyfriend came a few times. The other Lauren, from Annapolis, her husband, comes too. It's good to see their support."

"I wish more men saw the world like we do, Michael."

"Oh please," Michael said, brushing off his hands and then holding his palms up. "I'm an open book. I am what I am, and if somebody says, 'I don't like that,' then fine, I got more friends. I don't need you."

Michael became so comfortable sharing his life with others that he joined another support group at Karla's living facility. "Get this. They call that group Losing Your Marbles," he said, clapping his hands together. "There was another guy there too, and when I showed up, he said, 'Thank God you came here today. There are like ten other women and just me.'"

I wondered if their kids felt the same way because Michael was so transparent with Karla's condition. "What about the kids? Do they ever meet with someone?"

Michael loves talking about his children. "They love their mom, of course, but they also live outside Baltimore. Evan is the computer of the family—very techie, working on a start-up, and surfing around the world. First he worked in San Francisco and then in Seattle. He's visiting Karla's family in Brazil right now. He's fluent in Portuguese too. Elana was at college during all this, so they weren't home. It's easier to separate yourself when you're not there. And even now, they call me—because you can't call Karla—so they call me and they'll ask, 'How's mom?'"

Michael encourages his children to thrive while he holds down the care for Karla in Maryland. "Evan is all over the place with work, but Elana is a daddy's girl. We talk at least twice a day. Even when I'm in California, and she's in New York, we still call each other," Michael gushed.

"What does she do in New York?"

"Fashion merchandising," he said. "About five months ago, I took Karla to see Elana in New York. We saw some shows, and Elana was holding Karla's hand. Elana looked at Karla and said, 'Hey, Mom, you're doing great!'"

Even though their children don't visit Karla's living facility, Michael knows they always think about her. He doesn't get jealous when he sees other children or grandchildren there because everyone's case is different. However, Michael looks at the people he meets when visiting Karla as if they are his other family. Like the strangers you meet in therapy groups, you can't help but become close with people in the same position as you who are going through a life-changing milestone such as dementia.

"There was another woman I met there who had placed her husband at the living facility before I placed Karla. One day, she looks at me and says, 'So, how are you feeling? Are you feeling lonely, or are you feeling guilty?'"

Michael said her question was an ah-ha moment. "I started to tear up," he said. Then Michael put his hands on the table. "I said yes to both!"

"What was it like when you moved Karla in and had to say goodbye to her for that first night?" I asked.

Michael's eyes reddened with tears. He took off his glasses to wipe his face. His body language showed that their separation broke him into pieces, colored with hundreds of opposing feelings. There was guilt over leaving Karla, but there was also the confidence in knowing he was doing this because it was best for her. There was loneliness because she would never be with him in their house again, but relief in knowing he couldn't be selfish to keep her for his comfort. And, of course, there were the outside social voices that would play on repeat in Michael's mind, even though he tried to silence them with the security of knowing people looking on and wrongfully judging him would never really understand what life is like for him. Typically, he could care less about what outsiders think, just as long as his family knew Karla was being cared for.

"I notified her family, and they were very supportive. I said, 'Look, I have to do this for these reasons, but I will be there every day to see her.'" Michael still finds himself having to defend his decision. Fortunately, Karla's family knew and agreed that his decision was the best option for her. "They were all supportive. They're a great family."

When thinking about how close Michael has become with Karla's extensive Brazilian family, he told me about the first time he met all of them nearly forty years ago. From the first moment, he felt connected to her family. "There were only a handful of Jewish families in Manaus then, yet Karla's family had built the synagogue and the JCC. On the first night of Passover, all the Jewish families would go to the JCC and have a catered Passover dinner." Michael reiterated how well her family embraced him as if he had known them forever.

Michael waved his hand around as he spoke. "Karla was like, this is my cousin, this is my cousin, over here, this is my cousin. I said, 'I don't understand how you can have that many cousins?' But that's how it was," he said. "The Jewish families took care of the Jewish families, just as they did when I grew up and even now with our community. I loved it."

Having loved ones around Michael all the time became a natural development of his life. When the feeling of isolation began to seep through the cracks of dementia, Michael felt the burden of loneliness like never before. Throughout this book, I discuss the topic of isolation felt by those with dementia as well as care partners, which can drain the energy of everyone. Michael feels the sadness of isolation nearly every day. Like many others, it's also about companionship. Not romantic, but rather the connection of friendship.

Michael talked about connections throughout the breakfast, both personally and professionally. As a doctor, he made a career out of gaining people's trust as he performed eye surgeries, which was earned the hard way. Michael never felt alone regarding family, as he mentioned with Karla's extended "utopia in Brazil," as he called it, and the connections he made in Baltimore. The night of dropping off Karla at the living facility was the first time a life in solitude truly entered his mind.

Saying goodbye to Karla wasn't a cinematic send-off of two lovers kissing goodbye at the airport, knowing distance is the only thing between them. They were left with baggage to handle on their own. Michael cried more than he ever did when he left Karla. They would never be under the same roof again or be together to kiss each other goodnight. He'd miss her smile in the morning and her conversations over dinner, but most of all, he missed his best friend.

"What's something you miss from before?"

Michael shifted in his seat, crossed his legs, and scratched his head in thought. "Oh, the companionship," he said. "Now I see her as a patient—I don't see her as my companion. She'll hug me when I get there, but will she ask me how I feel. She goes, 'Oh, okay,' and that would be it. That would be our conversation. So I miss that. I miss her insight. We used to get together with her friends and talk so intelligently—not my friends, though," he added with a grin. "I miss that. I miss talking about politics. She lived in Israel, and I said to her, 'There's a war in Israel,' and she just replied, 'Oh, okay.' She lived in Israel for a while, and one of her brothers still lives in Israel and sent me a picture."

Talking about Israel and her family reminded Michael of other travels he wanted to do with Karla that he'd never been able to because of her condition. "One of my dreams was to go to Israel with her because she's fluent in Hebrew and has family there. We always talked about that. I want to go to Egypt. I want to go to Petra. I want to do all this!"

"Maybe you still can?"

Michael shrugged his shoulders. He knows he could but it wouldn't be the same without Karla. Even though he knows the rest of his life will be filled with moments that Karla won't be able to experience, Michael is still getting used to being alone. It's still a work in progress.

"I mean living by myself; I do everything alone. But there's a woman I have known for years whose husband passed away a while ago. We went to dinner a couple of times as friends," Michael said, pointing out the platonic companionship among care partners. "Another woman used to be a patient, and we have kept in touch ever since she moved away."

"It's better than dining alone," I said.

"Again, it's just either that or I watch TV while I eat dinner alone. These are people to talk to because the conversation with Karla is not a real conversation."

I needed Michael to know I would never judge him and hoped no one else would. "Michael, I don't think there's anything wrong with that. I think it's just humanistic about wanting to have an adult conversation with someone."

Michael nodded. Still, he knows many others won't feel the same way he and I do regarding companionship as a care partner. Sadly, having side-eye stares from people misjudging his life or having to explain his choices further is another detrimental part of dementia. Although Michael shared the downside effects of dementia, his upbeat humor convinced me he saw the beauty of keeping that Optimistic spirit.

"When you look at the disease though, Michael, are you— or how do you—stay optimistic?"

Michael looked past me as if his answer was floating behind me. "You do when you have some cognition. When you have supportive people who are going through what I'm going through while the rest of the world doesn't understand what I'm going through," he said. "I don't think anybody in our support group didn't come over to me and ask what they could do for me. They're good people, and that helps stay optimistic."

Following the topic of a positive support system, I asked, "What do you hope that people understand about this condition?"

"Well, the people living with it understand, but the rest of the world does not," he said. "You say, make a right turn, and they make a left. You get mad at them. You don't understand that it's not their fault. I hope that people could learn more about it and could say, there's no difference between cancer and this or asbestosis or mesothelioma. This wasn't a choice."

Michael was pointing to the idea that people seem to look at people with dementia as lost because there is no cure. The word alone is scary, and because there is no magic pill, people who have not experienced the world of dementia are too afraid to engage with people living with it. It's that concept that fuels Michael's mission to make Karla's story have a happy ending with all the love and support of her community.

After Michael and I left breakfast, I searched Manaus to understand where Karla was raised. I saw what her family had built, the legacy they left, and how the closeness of her family's commitment to one another allowed her community to expand. Manaus is colorful and majestic, overflowing with culture, music, and art. I also came across a Portuguese word, *saudade*, which holds many meanings. However, it's commonly defined as "the love that remains." It describes love and loss, passion and remorse, but most of all, its meaning provides hope. I wrote "saudade" on a sticky note and placed it on my desk, alongside other insights I gained from dozens of Optimistics I encountered during this journey. I looked at it as a reminder of my mission in honoring Karla's life and as a memento that hope is universal and admired by every culture around the globe in their unique way.

Today, Michael still sees patients and visits Karla every day. Although her health is declining, she has the best care imaginable for as long as she needs it. Michael still needs to check off any trips on his bucket list, but he's confident he will one day. For now, it's all about Karla, Evan, and Elana. When things don't make sense, Michael reveals that he and Karla built an incredible life together.

It's a far cry from the shy Jewish boy from Texas, who was frustratingly waiting at a bus stop outside Neiman Marcus and was moments away from finding his version of saudade. I hope Michael thanked his family for not taking him to the airport that day. After all, it worked out well for him in the end. Because for Karla and Michael, there is no end to their story, only saudade.

CHAPTER SEVEN

Dave and Kathy

HELLO, GORGEOUS

"**P**lanning for the future doesn't always work out the way you think it's going to," Kathy said, with a knowing grin to hide the darker meaning behind her statement.

To hear more about life with her late husband, Dave, aka "The Gentle Giant," I met Kathy at a restaurant in Baltimore called Stone Mill Bakery, on a warm summer morning, for coffee and breakfast.

Like many people from Maryland, Kathy and Dave grew up vacationing on the Delaware or Maryland shores, building lifelong memories in the sun. The summer after graduating college, Kathy and some friends rented the upstairs floor of a house in Rehoboth Beach, Delaware, for one more summer of freedom before the real world. At the same time, Dave shared the bottom floor with his family and friends. On paper, they seemed like opposites. Kathy was almost four years older, headed to a teaching position the fall. Dave was barely eighteen and his biggest worry was which bar to hang out on the beach that night. But, as they say, opposites attract.

"We came back to the beach house, and the guys were already passed out. We walked past them because Dave's room was actually the hallway under the stairs leading up to the girls area. And we see him sleeping there with his big red afro. I looked at my girlfriend and asked if we were staying with druggies. Dave's afro gave off that vibe."

That was Dave with the big red afro, and that's how Kathy first met him. That first summer, they became good friends but nothing else. After the summer ended, the two kept in touch and quickly realized something was developing between them. They ended up being married for thirty-seven years and had three kids.

At a YES group meeting, Kathy sat next to me by chance. She was a frequent visitor, but this was the first time we met. We connected right away. Kathy is petite, with short, bright gray hair, and was dressed in a refined red outfit. She looked as if she was about to give a presentation. On her wrists were silver bracelets and she had an elegant necklace on too. I point these things out because when I glanced at her, I noticed she had a tattoo on the inside of her forearm that seemed somewhat out of place for her current style.

"Excuse me, Kathy, but do you mind telling me what your tattoo says?"

"Sure! 'Hello, Gorgeous.' That's what Dave said to me every day. He never missed a day of answering the phone, 'Hello, Gorgeous.' Even if we were in the middle of the worst fight or disagreement or, you know, he always said '*Hello, Gorgeous*'–always."

I got chills.

"And that's his handwriting?"

"Yes. When he lost his ability to speak, he wrote it down, and I stuck it to the back of my phone so I could see it every day."

Kathy ran her hand over the tattoo as if touching her inked skin was also touching his skin.

"He was the opposite of me. He was a romantic, and I was the one who wasn't. I called him the big crybaby. He had a soft heart."

Being an emotional person like Dave, his ultimate desire was to care for his family, and for as long as he could, he tried to hide the effects of dementia. Dave built a career for himself, running his own business and being the provider for his family drove Dave to push forward. Ironically, Dave's business was the first victim of his disease.

To Dave's credit, he sacrificed his health to care for those who helped him build his business. "He tried to keep his guys employed. He was paying them rather than paying himself, that kind of thing, because he was a good person. But then we started noticing things happening. Money in the company wasn't where it was supposed to be."

"My oldest daughter is very pragmatic. She's the one who helped me to discover his speech issues because she worked for him at the time as his office manager. His business was going downhill. She's the one who came home from work and said, 'Mom, something's wrong with dad.' My middle daughter lived in Chicago, when she came home she noticed changes even more than we did seeing him every day"

Kathy's shoulders sank. "I said, you're confirming what I already suspected."

Dave's dementia took a sharp decline after he was diagnosed with Primary Progressive Aphasia, a type of frontotemporal dementia that affects someone's ability to speak. Dave went from talking normally to grunts and using a limited vocabulary of less than fifty words. In his later days, that number decreased to five or six at best. In the early years Dave could still hear and comprehend fairly well. Later, as the disease progressed, the frustration with his inability to verbally express himself only added to the fragile temperament most people with dementia can't control.

Even though he couldn't say, 'Hello, Gorgeous,' he and Kathy knew it was said in other ways.

Kathy showed me a video of Dave just a couple of months before his passing, revealing how he spoke. It was a language that could only be understood after thirty-seven years of marriage. Quickly after showing me that video, she showed me another video of a happier Dave.

"This is him and my son dancing in the kitchen. They're laughing!" In the video, Dave held hands with his son, dancing in the kitchen. Even though his body was deteriorating, as shown by his thin neckline, the smile on his face was pure happiness.

Kathy added, "This is maybe a month before he died, around December 11th, and he died January 17th."

Dave's situation is the cruel underbelly of dementia, showing no mercy when it comes to taking a person's life away. Not everyone gets to dance in the kitchen, and sadly, that was the last time Dave had ever held his son that way. I spoke to Kathy about the timetable of Dave's disease. Even though they knew they were fighting uphill, he continued to work and conduct his life as a contractor just as he did for decades before his diagnosis.

Like many people living with dementia, Dave didn't want to accept his fate and was determined to push the signs to the side to continue working. Although dementia forced him to close his business, he continued to do home repair and remodeling jobs for family and friends until his ability to measure and sequence a job was impaired.

"Six years in, he rebuilt my kitchen. He was defying the odds and we knew it."

Even though Dave could continue at least a portion of his career in a modified manner, by October of his final year, Dave had a minimal vocabulary of five or six words. The frustration of Dave's illness was taking more than just his ability to express himself properly. The disease caused tremendous mood swings in Dave, which became harder for Kathy to manage alone.

"We sold our house and had to downsize. It was too big for us. I wanted something more manageable. We moved into a townhouse. I became very close with the young couple who lived next door. I told them about Dave's condition and they were happy to help in any way they could."

Similar to other care partners' stories, the behaviors of people with dementia can be erratic and without cause. Parts of the brain that are important for reasoning, processing, and controlling emotions are damaged, making it almost impossible to verbally deescalate when someone is upset. Like a toddler throwing a tantrum, reasoning with Dave became incredibly difficult.

Kathy squirmed in her seat, adjusting to a part of her story that is the hardest part of the disease. "With the townhouse, our neighbors could hear everything going on. They heard Dave yelling at 2:00 AM or throwing items around. Once, he even painted our kitchen with a ketchup bottle."

As a result, Kathy's neighbor wanted to ensure Kathy was okay. "He would call me in the middle of the night when he could hear Dave going off the handle. He said, 'Look, bang on the wall, call me—I'll always leave my door unlocked—come running into my house, whatever you need,' because he knew that things were getting bad for me, that I was getting hurt."

Violent behavior is not uncommon in someone with dementia and is an unfair topic to discuss, yet Kathy handled it with grace. It wasn't Dave, her husband, who was out of control or who would growl uncontrollably. It was the disease taking over his body and adding a new reality to Kathy's home life. As Kathy knew, home would never be the same, and the townhouse held too many bad memories after he passed.

"I moved again to a condo. I couldn't stay in that house any longer—too many bad memories. I didn't want to live like that. I didn't want that house to be how I remembered Dave's last days."

"Did that change help you remain optimistic?" I asked.

During interviews for this book, everyone's response to that question garnered a different reaction. Knowing that it can make some people cry or reflect on something more philosophical, they feel they owe me. I wanted to let Kathy understand I sympathize with having to conjure an answer to a question she did not focus on before meeting me.

I told Kathy, "The thing that's fascinating about optimism is it's different for everyone. Look, I'm not a very religious person. I'm Jewish and I love being Jewish but I don't go to synagogue. I do it my way."

Then, I pointed to a small Buddha sculpture, alongside plants on the shelf behind Kathy. "Look, there's Buddha right there. I think he's awesome! I mean, whatever entity comes in, I'm happy with whatever someone chooses."

Kathy laughed.

"But, I'm also not an 'everything happens for a reason' kind of guy," I add.

"No!" Kathy cheered. "If I tried to say that to myself, I'd be pissed off. I hate that saying because, really, what did I do that deserved this? What did my kids do that deserved this? There is nothing. What reason could you possibly have? I hate that saying."

"I'm with you," I energetically replied.

Kathy followed up her disdain for that by saying, "People who say that have never had something terrible happen. Or not terrible enough."

"I'm with you," I energetically replied.

Kathy followed up her disdain for that by saying, "People who say that have clearly never had something terrible happen to them. Or not terrible enough to make it worth not being like, 'Fuck this, I can't believe this!'" she shouted to me.

Kathy's free-flowing language is a good sign that she's getting to the nature of optimism in her way, as everyone in her position should. You don't always get to choose what things happen to you, but you do control how you handle them. I wanted Kathy to know that being optimistic is a challenge, even for "Mr. Optimistic," as she jokingly called me.

"Kathy, I don't know how I would stay optimistic."

"First of all, nobody's optimistic 100% of the time. Everybody goes through bouts of anger and depression. But I think what keeps you optimistic, or what kept me optimistic, was, if I live on the black side of this, then I will have no fond memories of the last ten years."

My ears perked, and my heart dropped when she mentioned the black side of her story because that is the struggle for anyone who has to watch a loved one pass away in front of their eyes.

"I have wonderful memories of when we were younger."

"Including the red afro?" I asked.

"Including the red afro!" She laughs, then continues, "I didn't want all my memories of him to only be from that time. I wanted to have memories during this time that showed me he was still here. We still had a good time from time to time. We still had to laugh, we still understood each other. He still loved me, and I still loved him. That came from finding something to smile about every day and laugh at—even if we were laughing at him and not with him, we were still laughing."

I agreed, "Laughter definitely helps in remaining optimistic."

"I think you stay optimistic because what choice do you have besides falling into the blackness of it and not being able to crawl out?"

Blackness is a theme with care partners and those who have dementia. The fragility that comes with isolation and confusion stirs up dark emotions that battle for your time.

Sadly, the hole that dementia digs grows larger every day and makes the ability to keep crawling that much more challenging. However, as Kathy said, only *you* can choose to lift yourself out.

"That was my fear. I felt if I succumbed to the horrible, overwhelming feeling that life was over, I would not climb out myself. I knew that would be easy to do. I could have fallen into that black pit very easily and stayed there. I'd rather battle to be optimistic than give up."

"Not many people can climb out like you did," I said.

"Because you fight it, you become optimistic. The only way to fight it is to find something to be optimistic about. You have to find something to smile about, something to be happy about, something to love."

Love, hope, and strength kept Kathy and Dave together for so long, and it was their love that she turned to in his final days. Dave's illness grew quicker towards the end, and before she knew it, he was lying in a medically induced coma in hospice. Kathy didn't need a reminder to know what hospice meant for him.

"When we arrived, the doctors said it could be three or four weeks, but I knew otherwise."

Dave lasted only six days.

Determined to make sure his final days were filled with love, even in a coma, Kathy never left Dave's side. Family and friends came in to say their goodbyes and to comfort Kathy. On Dave's last morning, his heart rate went up to 121 beats per minute, and his body had taken all the nutrition out of his muscles, leaving a frail reflection. The nurses told Kathy today was the day.

Upon hearing that news, the blackness seeped back into Kathy's heart, positioning for dominance over the last spots reserved for Dave. Although Kathy had anticipated this day coming, she never truly knew what to expect. You can think about your loved one's final days and imagine what you would say, but you never know until that day is presented without warning.

However, the one thing Kathy did know was how she wanted Dave's last days to go, and it wasn't about taking a last breath alone. She lay next to Dave in his bed. With the nurses' help, they draped Dave's marionette arms over Kathy. She stared at his face, watching his fragile mouth take smaller and smaller breaths. Kathy said her final words to Dave. She spoke of forgiveness and love and thanked him for being an amazing partner. Dave could not respond, but Kathy knew he was at peace.

Dementia may have stolen much from Kathy and Dave, but their lives were not solely those years. Kathy brushed her teary fingers across his cheeks. At that moment, Dave's condition and the past several years vanished. They were two just kids at the beach discovering adulthood, dancing on the sand, and holding each other under the stars. Dave's hair wasn't thin and brittle but rather thick and dusty from the sand. He wasn't silent but instead filled with the same passion he displayed every day with Kathy.

Somewhere in their embrace, Dave said, *'Hello, Gorgeous'* and somehow Kathy heard it.

On January 17, 2023, at 10:40 AM David Charles Rogers took his final breath.

He was fifty-eight.

CHAPTER EIGHT

Mark and Evie

EVIE AND THE FROZEN ORANGE

*"Therefore I tell you, whatever you ask in prayer, believe that you have received it, and it will be yours." —*Mark 11:24

Every single person with Alzheimer's Dementia asks, "Why me?" A fair question for a disease that has no rhyme or reason as to who it attacks. Some people deal with it better than others. Whether it's through family, therapy, religion, or just settling on accepting their diagnosis, the why is never truly answered.

After I came across Evie's husband, Mark, who dedicated his life to God as a Pastor, I was curious to hear how Mark, a man of faith, addressed the "why" debate.

When I first met Evie, her sunny demeanor radiated from her wide smile and sensitive eyes behind her glasses. She's talkative yet soft-spoken at the same time, almost therapeutically. In the YES group meetings, Evie operates not only as a facilitator but also offers a wealth of knowledge to care partners. After Mark's diagnosis, she dedicated her life to studying the dementia that would eventually steal her husband.

Similar to the world of faith, Evie committed herself to the world of care, not only for Mark but also for others who would surpass his life. Like almost every care partner with dementia, she had her faith tested, tried, and, at times, conflicted. Despite his condition, Mark answered the challenge with the word of God. He was called to service, and serving was what he would do until his dementia worsened.

The Optimistics told me that life is split into two eras: the time before the diagnosis and then the time after. Like a neon light, the words, "Yes, you have dementia," blinds your eyes into believing there is no other answer. Yet, while many of those with ADRD search for their new purpose, Mark always knew his mission was to connect with others in his position.

When Evie asked her husband what he wanted to do, he said, "I'm still called to ministry." That was Mark. Like most people of faith, he committed his entire life to God. In his eyes, dementia would not interfere with God's plan.

Mark went to college in Michigan for two years, during which time his parents were going through a divorce, which had a life-changing impact on him and his teenage sister. Mark had always treated his role of big brother as more of a father figure since their father was somewhat absent. He took his parent's divorce as a more profound reason to challenge his faith. Providing service through faith was what Mark would do until he no longer could.

He still had work to do, and like any true showman, it was hard to let the audience down. He not only looked like the part of a pastor, but his charisma and presentation captivated his audience. Mark loved working on his sermons and dissecting the bible's teachings as his tool to illustrate the reasons for certain aspects of life that needed his inspirational voice.

"Mark was a very vital speaker," she began. "Many people would tell me, 'When he preached, I knew he was talking right to me,'" she added with a proud grin.

When you make your life on a stage, you welcome eyes on you at all times, whether praise or scrutiny. Over time, those eyes who looked to Mark for guidance started to look at one another in concern. The church's apprehension would soon become gossip, and Mark needed a break.

"I remember Mark was at church one night. It was still Saturday, and he spent all day Saturday writing; however, he was still there until about 10:00 at night. And it's like, what is up with that?"

Mark told Evie he couldn't bring it together and needed more time, which was not Mark's style. Even the next morning, he was struggling. The murmurs in the congregation began to increase.

"Our denomination has a board, and I think Mark's executive skills were compromising his leadership. There was some restlessness going on with the board. Then some people started leaving."

Along with church members parting ways with Mark, so did the community around him and Evie. The members needed their leader, and it was clear that Mark was losing their trust.

Call it ego or embarrassment, he did not reveal his fears about his lessening abilities. As I found with every person I met, the idea that their professional life, which they've worked tirelessly for decades to enhance, is no longer their purpose was the most challenging aspect of dementia to accept. By default, being the pastor's wife represents their spouse's passion for the church. You get the glory when it's good and the negativity when it's bad.

Eventually, the board decided Mark was no longer suitable for the job and he stepped down. To add salt to Mark's wound and rebuild the church, Mark and Evie had to distance themselves completely, including from friends they had made. This concept isn't new to clergy. You must allow them to build their practice out of respect for the new pastor.

Once again, the themes of loss, isolation, and your new life after a diagnosis were brought to the surface. Mark went from having hundreds of people listen to his every word and be moved with passion to sitting idle in his living room as Evie looked on.

She recalled the first days of Mark's new life with both frustration and angst. That was not how his final days at the church should have gone. The Showman doesn't get yanked off stage; they get a curtain call of applause in front of a crowd.

"There's no comprehension of how you interpret this change in your life. Because if you're retiring, I guess you become uncalled when you retire. And it's just..." Evie creased her lips, then said, "It was too soon. For Mark, it was, 'Who am I now?' He said, 'I'm still called to ministry, so now what do I do?'"

Despite it all, Mark never lost his faith or doubted God.

"Mark and I never believed that people of faith are protected from harm. We pray for that, but we're not protected from disease. There are plenty of pastors and religious faith-based people who pass at a young age. Tragedy and suffering exist in the world. God is in the suffering with us. Initially, people experiencing hardships gets stuck in the "Why, God?" question." But as Mark came out of the shock of the diagnosis, he focused on making himself available to help and serve to hers in this unexpected world of dementia."

Even though Mark's optimism in still practicing was a sign of encouragement, she knew her job was to show him how to remain focused on his calling. She knew it wouldn't be as easy as simply believing it would take action.

*   *   *   *   *

Evie and Mark settled into their new life. Mark's absence at the church was felt not only amongst the congregation but also in their house. Evie watched Mark go from capturing the emotions of hundreds with his original sermons to sitting idle on their living room couch reading a book without comprehension.. They couldn't live like this, she thought. Mark still had a calling, and it was not to live his final years away from others he could impact.

An educational support meeting held at Frederick County Senior Services reached out to Evie about discussing Alzheimer's Dementia and how Mark was coping. The room was filled with individuals with dementia and care partners of all ages sitting at round tables. Mark was at the table next to Evie by the podium. She had her notes and a plan, but that washed away with a flow of open dialogue from a place she had kept hidden from many. Evie spoke about Mark with pride, love, and admiration. Halfway through her speech, a hand shot up from one of the round tables.

"That's me! That's me she's talking about." It was Mark.

Evie remembers that day as a glimpse into who Mark once was. "Then he patted his chest, like 'That's me!' Then this other woman who was a little older, she and her husband were at another table, but she said, 'Yes, that's me too!'"

He walked over to the woman and knelt beside her. He put his hand on her shoulder and looked into her gentle eyes.

"Although I don't know what he said, he said something to her. I couldn't hear, but I just started to tear up because... there's Mark being Mark. One caregiver came up to me and he said, 'You can take him out of the church, but you can't take the pastor out of him.'"

Mark was still impassioned to walk alongside others.

That was a day that Evie kept in the part of her brain reserved only for the good days. Mark's openness and ability to touch new people like he did in the past was only a cruel tease, convincing her there would be many more days like this, to outweigh his illness. Good days like that were moments that became fewer and farther apart. Mark became more agitated and solitary. Friends found it hard to engage with her and Mark, which amplified the feeling of isolation. One morning, she was determined to chase a memorable day. They planned to attend a community concert and get Mark some needed social outreach. The rain poured heavier than it had in weeks, which normally Evie wouldn't risk.

"But did I stay home? No. No, we're going to go do something physical and social," she said with defiance. "We went out with our rain jackets and umbrellas, and the concert ended up being canceled." Evie tilted her head as if to say, "Of course it is!"

"Mark was so miserable. His face was all scrunched up and he was not happy. But we're standing on this bridge, in the rain, and I took a picture because I thought, this is so ridiculous what I'm doing," she laughed.

Evie still has the photo today.

Mark's unhappiness with the littlest of things began to take over every aspect of their lives. Even though she fought for the slightest moment of normalcy, Mark's aggression grew out of control with nervous agitation and false narratives. Evie was running out of options until she heard about the frozen orange technique. This idea came from their son, Aaron, who is a Clinical Social Worker and the Program Director of a residential treatment program for individuals with severe and persistent mental illnesses.

"Aaron said, put an orange in the freezer. When Mark is getting a distorted reality, you try to bring him back into what's right there in front of you—like get grounded."

Evie would hold Mark's hand in hers with the frozen orange between them, trying to nurture his mind to some sense of reality. She would drill him with questions to distract him. "What does the orange feel like? Is it cold? Why is it cold? Is it soft or hard?"

Frozen orange moments turned into frozen orange days.

During one difficult day, Evie took Mark for a drive down a back country road, which he normally enjoyed and usually calmed him down. They would listen to music and then stop for pizza, hoping to create another moment for themselves. However, that did not work out as planned. On the way back to the car, Mark became agitated and confused about his surroundings. He didn't understand how to open the car door.

His brain was telling him to fight and he began kicking the side of the rear door of their car, to the point he was trying to thrust his foot through the door. Evie opened it for him and he slumped into the backseat with defiance.

"I thought he would enjoy music in the car, but he was restless and agitated. Nothing was making sense to him, and he couldn't clarify enough to help and figure it out."

In Mark's mind, he was trapped and even betrayed.

"I'm still thinking I can create an environment that calms him down. You know, distract him with the peaceful lanes of farm life. But, I think he was worried that I was taking him to assisted living."

Shortly after, Mark took off his size twelve sandal and threw it at her head, while she was driving. Finally, Evie had enough. This would be a moment to remember, but not a picture worth keeping. She pulled over to the shoulder and scolded Mark, hoping that would rattle him from the tantrum. Evie opened the car, leaned against the hood, and cried.

Mark's delusions increased to the point she could not combat his strength. On more than one occasion, their son, Aaron had to wrestle his dad into compliance. On a visit to Aaron's house, Evie left Mark alone which she believed led to panic. Mark opened the dining room window and tried to jump out. Although it was not far to the ground, in his state, it was still a fall. Aaron had to use force to contain him. On another occasion, Mark took a bottle of pills and dared Aaron to stop him from swallowing all of them. Again, Aaron had to physically control his father. Instances like that made it clear that Mark needed more assistance than Evie could manage. She had avoided this step because she knew what it meant.

"You know that once they leave home, they're not coming back," she said, implying the inevitable.

*   *   *   *   *

Aaron

After Evie and I spoke, I was curious about her children's take on Mark's illness and how they viewed optimism. I connected with their son, Aaron who, similar to Mark, has spent his entire professional life dedicated to helping others in need. One thing they didn't teach Aaron in school was how to handle your father fighting you as if attacked by a stranger in the night.

"I had been used to compartmentalizing a lot of things in life anyway, working in juvenile facilities or working in residential mental health. It's not my first time tackling someone who's trying to hurt me or someone else. But with my dad, I would try to keep him from running away or him from trying to hit me to prevent him from hurting himself or someone else. It's confusing to try to figure out what level of force it takes to do that."

Mark was over six feet tall and two hundred pounds at his healthiest. Aaron, a former rugby player, inherited his father's build, along with the deep baritone of a radio announcer. Aaron's face; however, was Evie's. When he popped onto my screen, I saw Evie in his eyes, smile, and the kind demeanor she handed down. Like Mark, Aaron knows how to make people feel comfortable, and from the moment we began talking, I immediately felt close to him, like I did with

Evie. Aaron began to see signs in Mark that seemed out of character. He described those moments as the initial part of his journey with his dad's illness.

"I think we had our suspicions for a long time. I remember this journey for us starting back in 2008. Back then we started seeing cognitive issues; like forgetting things, misplacing things, having a hard time, and doing some of the sequencing work—common cognitive functions that we all do on a day-to-day basis."

Being a seasoned therapist, Aaron knew how to read people. He uncovers what people may be hiding by watching their actions and interactions. With dementia, everyone is hiding something because they want to believe the world can't tell. Aaron could have held that view. However, having seen this in others throughout his career, he had a realistic—and scary—view of what was to come. That knowledge tipped the scale for Aaron wanting to move back home to Fredrick to help his mom with Mark's care.

Aaron knew there was no way to stop Mark's decline but as he said, "Now you're treating the ripples from the actual thing. We're not dealing with just Alzheimer's now."

Uncovering what Mark would be facing from a medical standpoint was what Aaron prepared himself for; however, his role in the house came with several hats. First and foremost, Aaron was a son. His main focus was to do what was needed for his parents. His wife and young son were on board. Sometimes, Aaron was a marital therapist, acting as a soundboard for the frustrations that dementia causes in marriages. Around the clock, he used his medical background to monitor Mark and work with Evie to make sense of new developments, especially when there were declines in Mark's health. While navigating this, with sporadic roadblocks the disease presented, Aaron always made time to find father-son moments with his dad.

I asked him if Mark understood what was happening as things got worse and if Aaron had to explain Mark's condition to him. Aaron looked off smiling and laughed, thinking of Mark at the house, especially on their many bonding times sitting on the couch together. Quickly though, Aaron's tone changed and his eyes watered. The smile was in honor of Mark's ability to always think of his family first, even when it was Mark's needs that should be considered primary.

"We'd sit on the couch and he knew that he was cognitively going. He knew that he wouldn't be around forever. He was always someone who wanted to take care of and protect people. He did everything around the house for everybody. The kind of person who always showed up."

Aaron wiped his tears with his palms as he opened up further.

"But that time he was really worried about the future. We'd sit on the couch, we'd hold hands, and he would just repeat," Aaron began, with his deep voice getting muffled with emotion, "He would repeat, 'Just take care of Mom. Just take care of Mom. Just take care of Mom.'"

Aaron held Mark's hand tighter and assured Mark. "I'd promise him I'd do that and say, 'Of course, I always have and always will.'"

Over time, Aaron's commitment to Evie's safety had to be shown with physicality, rather than nurture. He began to take over his understanding of the future, solely focused on the present, as his mind tortured his body into disbelief.

"I would try to verbally deescalate, then push away, and be like, 'What are we doing, man?' Then it's using all the emotional tools to say, 'It's me, Dad. This is me. I don't know why we're trying to fight.' It's this weird duality of trying to protect yourself and him while trying to form this emotional connection and bond. Those were weird moments."

"When those moments happened and you reminded him of things, did it bring him back or did it calm him down?" I asked.

"Both have been true. There were times when I would bear hug or judo hold him on the ground for maybe twenty minutes of him fighting. He's trying to use all of his old man strength to get away, while I'm on his back for twenty minutes. It was exhausting."

While Mark's brain struggled to free himself, Aaron continued to try and connect with Mark despite the mental and physical struggle neither man envisioned happening as father and son. Aaron tried to take himself out of the conflict. He closed his eyes, and balanced his strength, not meant to hurt his father. Both men panting and sweating, while Aaron whispered into Mark's ears, "I love you."

"As I'm holding him down, I would just keep saying to him, 'I love you, I love you,' over and over."

Moments like that pale in comparison to the admiration he had for Mark. Even though he wasn't the man he grew up with, he was still his father, and still a man of faith with a calling. Mark's actions weren't his fault. Afterward, he had no recollection of the altercations. Aaron had to keep reminding himself of that, despite the agony it caused them. Aaron also could never go back on his promise to always take care of his mom. Part of the mother-son commitment involved Mark being placed into a assisted living facility, where he could be tended to around the clock.

Aaron remembers vividly the time he spent with Mark while he lived there and was astonished at how his father continued operating by his faith.

"It took a long time for him to accept people doing everything for him. Even till the very end, he would be a proud man who would try to do as much as he could. I mean, even in the assisted living facility, which was only the last three months of his life, he would still have a Bible and try to pray for people and meet with people and do pastoral counseling there."

The proud moments of Mark's calling while at the assisted living facility helped him further accept where he lived, and also accept knowing he would not go home. Aaron got the most emotional during this part of our discussion because it involved his son, Ezekiel (Zeke), and his relationship with his grandfather.

"I remember the day Dad went into the assisted living facility and I brought my oldest son, Zeke, who was about a year and a half old. We're walking in and Zeke grabs Dad's hand and walks him inside. Dad grabs it back."

As a father of two, I couldn't imagine the thought process of any toddler, let alone that young, handling an emotion like that.

"At only a year and a half?" My eyes widened.

"Zeke was already smarter than me then," Aaron joked.

"We have this picture. Zeke almost knew, 'Hey, Grandpa needs help', and then Grandpa accepted that as he's walking in."

Aaron shook his head as if still in the moment, dabbing his eyes dry with his hand. "It's such a beautiful, beautiful picture. Both of them love the relationship they had."

As I do with everyone, I wanted to see how he viewed optimism with Mark. Did the change in Mark's personality fog Aaron's viewpoint on how he looked at optimism in the face of dementia?

"When it comes to optimism for me, it's having the luxury of having that perspective for a lot of my life in the last fifteen years. Those feel like luxuries because there's a lot of these hard moments. With Dad, it's like you're in trench warfare. All you're thinking about is, 'How do I get through today and how do I manage this next outburst or how do I manage the problems that he's experiencing?' I was so hyper-focused on the minutiae and you need to be able to create space for perspective. You know, go home that night and think, what a hard day—but that time Dad laughed, like that, oh man, that was a good moment."

Like Evie, Aaron capsulized his time with Mark into moments that only clarity and perspective could digest.

* * * * *

Mark's final days were bedridden but surrounded by friends and family. Each day they thought was his last, a community of visitors allowed Mark to rally for another day. His speech was limited but he knew what was happening and felt the comfort of his loved ones.

Evie recalled the time one visitor came to see Mark who she had never met, but it was clear that she and mark Mark had a connection.

"I remember there was this young girl, she was in her early twenties, and there had been an awful family situation that Mark had gotten involved in. She had driven a long distance, but the message she wanted to give Mark, and she kept saying it over and over again, 'Mark, you saved my family.'"

Mark didn't have to say a word to show his gratitude for her. Although their interaction was non-verbal, the young woman knew Mark had the same compassion for her now as he did in the past.

"I could just see that eye contact was there and he was definitely engaged and kind of receiving the love. He was beautiful."

The remainder of Mark's life was spent with Evie and his children by his bedside. They held his hands, read prayers, sang songs, and reminded Mark that Jesus awaited him. At this point, Mark's body disintegrated into a skeletal shell of the broad-shouldered man he once was but he was still the pastor who commanded attention. Dementia took his mind first, then chipped away at his body, but his soul was still healthy. Inside Mark's body, the family knew in confidence that he was watching over them.

The last words to a loved one are tedious on the heart, and Evie and her boys had their messages to share with Mark. Aaron told me that when he sat with his dad, he wanted his dad to know how proud he was of him, and that everyone would be okay, especially Evie.

About the final words he spoke to Mark, Aaron said, "I just wanted to say those things. I know he may not be hearing it, but I couldn't live with myself for not saying it."

Evie spoke of faith and heaven. She thought only of the precious moments they had together and the husband, father, and best friend he was to her. As she held Mark's hand, she waited for the final breaths to leave Mark's body. Evie didn't need a camera for this memory. She had already prepared herself for this day that would forever live in her heart.

Only three days before Christmas, on December 22, 2018, with his family by his side, Reverend Mark Henry VanderMeer was called upon to the Lord one last time. He was sixty-five.

CHAPTER NINE

Katherine and Sarah

HUGGING COWS AND OTHER DREAMS

66 There are moments where I can just see that she'll have pure joy moments and moments where it's hard when she'll forget certain things. But when it is a happy moment, it's like a real happy moment because it's like the first time she's hearing it."

Strength and dignity don't even begin to describe the story of Sarah and Katherine. I've met dozens of spouses who have endured the pain of watching their partner battle with dementia and seen adult children take on the parental role. However, I've never met someone fresh out of college who has to be the only care partner for their mother.

If life after college isn't stressful enough with managing work, bills, and real-life drama that tests your limitations, try taking on the sole responsibility of becoming your parent's parent. This happened to twenty-five-year-old Sarah Close, who became Katherine's mother and guardian.

Sarah calls herself a grandma stuck in a twenty-something's body. Unlike most young adults who spend their weekends in bars, Sarah goes antiquing at flea markets. She skipped the fancy restaurants on her birthday this year. Instead, she settled for a local home and garden show. While other kids her age are surfing dating apps, Sarah enjoys spending time with her rescue dog, Milo, and playing Disney trivia with her friends. But even being an old soul does not mean one is designed to handle the weight of adulthood responsibilities outside of themselves. Sarah said, "I had to become a mom for my mom."

Being shot into the role of parenthood changes nearly every aspect of a typical young adulthood lifestyle. Sarah knew her situation was vastly different from others her age.

"Friends, like their understanding? I guess they don't know what to do. They're kind of like, 'Oh, I had a grandparent that had dementia' or stuff like that. They don't know how to respond."

I am guilty of this as well. My only relationship with dementia before writing this book was with my grandmother and other elderly family members. Before I met the Optimistics, at forty-four, I was unaware that Young-Onset Dementia could happen to someone at my age, and I found that I wasn't alone in my naivete. Plus, Sarah's right. People don't get what it's like for her, which can only add to the isolation that ADRD, like Vascular Dementia, bring to those who carry its weight. Sarah would eventually find that what she had to bear was heavier than she imagined and would take a darker turn in how it got lighter.

*　　　*　　　*　　　*　　　*

Katherine, who also has multiple sclerosis (MS), began to show signs of dementia during the pandemic's lockdown stage. With many assisted living and therapy facilities closed during COVID-19, Sarah moved into her mother's apartment. At that time, Kathy's nerves became more delicate, and paranoia consumed her. Although capable of living independently with her MS, Kathy had not yet been diagnosed with dementia. Her outbursts and anxiety were signs of what would come, but nothing like Sarah would imagine.

Having started a new job as a preschool teacher, Sarah rented a townhouse with a friend. She needed to be a real adult, and gaining independence was only part of her reason for leaving. The more critical matter surrounded Kathy's worsening health during the pandemic. MS is an autoimmune disease, and the last thing Sarah wanted was to bring COVID-19 into Kathy's close quarters.

Sarah remained close to Kathy during this time, but with each visit, Sarah noticed something new that elevated Kathy's anxiety. Her quirky habits became less moderate and grew to the extreme. Kathy refused to take her garbage out to the apartment trash facility. She was also too nervous to do her laundry in the community laundry room because strangers in her building scared her. On one visit, Sarah saw dozens of trash bags sitting in Kathy's apartment. She was also terrified of the grocery store and, as a result, had a bare fridge. Kathy only ate junk food from the 7-11 across the street, where she would also grab packs of cigarettes.

Sarah's visits turned into errand running, doing Kathy's laundry, taking out extensive collections of trash, and providing healthier grocery shopping. Kathy's fears turned into hallucinations and delusions, which was a sign of her vascular dementia.

She complained to Sarah that "creatures" were living in her apartment. These creatures were to blame for the trash piling up in the kitchen. Sarah assumed what her mom saw were mice. Even though an exterminator found nothing wrong, Kathy was convinced something was in her apartment. She pointed to coffee grains on the table, which she likely dropped herself, as signs of the creatures invading her space. In severe instances, Kathy hid garbage in the refrigerator or placed cups and mugs in her microwave. She was hiding them so the creatures could not get to them.

Sarah did her best to calm her mom from the falsehoods her eyes were showing her, but that didn't stop Kathy from complaining to the apartment manager. After several visits from the apartment manager, Kathy yelled at him and blamed him for the creatures still ruining her home. Eventually, the manager wrote Kathy off as crazy and ignored her calls. While the apartment staff separated themselves from Kathy, her mind continued to unravel into a world of her own due to her uncontrollable paranoia.

"My mom was going to put bleach water out to kill the creatures, forgetting about her cat, Gracie. And I was like, 'Mom, you can't do that!'" Sarah said, remembering the day she stepped in to remove Kathy from the apartment.

Kathy was very unhealthy by this time, and her body showed it. When Sarah confronted her mom about her health, Kathy couldn't realize her current state. With no defined answers to her mom's bizarre behavior, Sarah figured Kathy's crippling paranoia was a side effect of her troubled past. Outside of the pain Kathy felt from her MS, she battled depression for decades, amplified by the death of her late husband years prior.

The day after New Year's, Kathy's husband—Sarah's stepfather—shot himself in the parking lot of a food store while Kathy was sitting in the passenger seat of their car. That moment shattered their worlds. Even though he was her parent through marriage, Sarah had always looked at her stepfather as her real father. She believes Kathy never reconciled his death, which added to the cocktail of pain her mind was put through. She drank heavier, smoked more, and did what she could to relieve her mind from that agony. Nothing worked. Like the bags of trash speckled around Kathy's apartment, her mental health found pockets of its own to waste away. Sarah realized she needed to move her mom again to keep Kathy safe.

Talks about moving made Sarah the most emotional during our discussion. Since every move Kathy made was to a smaller place, that meant less room for the life they built as a mother and daughter. Sarah took a moment to pause and collect herself, but that did not stop her tears.

"We can take a break if you like," I said.

She patted her eyes dry. "No, I'm fine, I'm fine," Sarah said. "Sorry," she added, taking a breath. "Okay. When I moved her, it hit me that I won't be able to go home anymore. It hit me hard that I had to get rid of a lot of my old kid stuff."

Sarah eventually switched jobs and became a paraeducator and donated the toys to her school. However, other more personal items were simply tossed away without a care. Yearbooks, photographs, and the memorable accessories that adorned her wall for years no longer interested Kathy. Item after item, Sarah asked, "Why?" Kathy would say she didn't even remember the people in the photos, as if she had framed memories of strangers. With every memory Kathy placed into the trash pile, Sarah felt her mom float farther and farther away from her past.

Moving from the apartment to the studio meant Sarah would no longer have a home. As disorganized as the apartment was, Sarah had a bed and a place where she could stay with Kathy. In the studio, Sarah would only be a visitor. Box after box of Kathy's past was sent to the dumpster, leaving Sarah with a newfound level of emptiness when she stared back at what remained. Not only did vascular dementia take away Kathy's true mind, but it also convinced her to disregard her past.

"In the end, I had five tubs of items. That's all my mom has to her name, five tubs."

The downsizing of Kathy's home reflected her state at the time: confined, isolated, and small. After Kathy settled in, Sarah thought a minimal lifestyle would make her life more manageable. Regardless of how little Kathy had, her mental health concerns continued to crowd her life.

At her new home, Sarah got calls from Kathy at all hours complaining about gangs following her around, tapping her phone, and even planning an attack. Sarah tried to reason with Kathy about how ludicrous the idea of anyone doing these things to her, but Kathy wouldn't flinch in her beliefs. Sarah tried to talk sense into Kathy by asking why the gangs would care about her, hoping to make sense of that absurdity. Kathy couldn't be swayed. She was adamant that gangs were out to get her. After only a few months, Sarah was forced to admit Kathy to a hospital for further evaluation.

The months passed, and Sarah, only twenty-five at the time, continued to operate as her mother's keeper. She paid her bills, cleaned the studio, and answered her mail. As Christmas approached, it was clear that Kathy would not come home in time to celebrate as they did years before. Still, Sarah kept the meaning of family for the holidays the best way she could.

"We had our own Christmas in the hospital. I made her some Polish snowflakes, which was a tradition, and she hung them up in her little room. She felt bad she couldn't buy me anything because she was in the hospital, but she drew me a picture. It was so sweet."

Two days after Christmas, while still in the psychiatric hospital, Kathy fell. She hit her head, blacked out, and broke her femur. She was transported to a different hospital so they could perform surgery to repair the break. Kathy refused to get the surgery because she thought the doctors were going to put a microchip in her. If she didn't get the surgery she would not be able to walk again. Since she was deemed not of sound mind with no official power of attorney on record, being her next of kin, Sarah had to decide on her mother's behalf about the surgery. This was the first official decision that Sarah had to make on behalf of her mother. After her surgery, the doctors performed further cognitive testing which is when they concluded that she had vascular dementia.

*   *   *   *   *

Weeks later, while going through some of Kathy's old paperwork, Sarah found what she thought would be a lifeline to aid in Kathy's care. There were documents indicating a power of attorney involving her aunt. Finally, Sarah had in writing who could assist with major decisions involving Kathy. It named a much older, more experienced adult. Unfortunately, Sarah's aunt wanted no part in managing Kathy's life, nor did Kathy's other sister.

Sarah was once again the only one left to fend for Kathy.

"I felt heartbroken. One, my aunt didn't want to do it, and then I felt like oh, I'm a parent now."

Adulthood took on a greater meaning than it did for Sarah's friends, who couldn't quite handle the state of Kathy. Sarah accepted that her version of her twenties wouldn't be filled with happy hours and weekends with kids her age. She took on all secretarial and managerial duties for her mom. She had to schedule Kathy's appointments, balance their finances, and oversee her mom's growing legal issues.

"How were you able to just take this on?" I asked in wonder, seeing as I could never do the same if I were in her position.

Sarah shook her head. "I didn't know where anything was. I didn't know where the title to her car was, I didn't know this stuff! And at the same time, I'm trying to get my own life together."

With no other help from Kathy's sisters and no official legal dominion over Kathy, Sarah either had to make her case to take over as Kathy's guardian or allow the state to take over. The latter would mean that Sarah would lose all ability to assist Kathy or have a say in her well-being.

Sarah was only twenty-five at the time.

To make her claim known, she had to follow the proper legal procedures to stop the state from getting involved. During a video court hearing, Sarah and her pro-bono lawyer faced a judge and Kathy's sisters. Her aunts had to use this time as their opportunity to relinquish their power of attorney over Kathy. Sarah watched her aunts, who kept avoiding eye contact with her. She felt betrayed. Even worse, Kathy did not have to be present for the hearing, which made her sisters' cowardly and pathetic excuses easier to slide past the judge.

Kathy's sisters pleaded their case for not being able to care for Kathy. Then Sarah, as the last, most suitable option, had to declare her intent.

"My aunts had to present and say that they felt I was suitable to be the guardian. Then, it was my turn to show I was good enough for it."

Due to Maryland state law, there had to be a legal defense against Sarah's petition for guardianship. A court-appointed lawyer, who had never met Kathy or Sarah, made a case against Sarah's abilities. Had Sarah been in her forties, this would have been a no-brainer, but because she was thrust into this role at twenty-five, her age was the only hindrance in her case.

Finally, after Sarah finished wiping away her tears in front of the court, the judge awarded Sarah full guardianship. However, after the court made it official, Sarah only had six days to find her mom in an assisted living facility other than the hospital.

"I had no idea where to begin. Thankfully, one of the counselors laid out three options based upon my mom's financial situation."

Of all the options they could afford, a home-based care facility, where Kathy would likely have a room in someone's house, was an ideal option. Sarah chose the best location and then moved her mom to another home. Kathy only had two trash bags filled with clothes and personal items while she was at the geriatric psych hospital. However, when Sarah arrived to move Kathy to her new assisted living facility, those bags were missing.

"How? Did someone rob her?"

"I don't know," Sarah said, shaking her head. "But when we left, she only had two shirts and the pants she was wearing. She didn't even have shoes!"

Sarah had built up a solid resilience for people's intolerance towards her mother that she didn't even care to battle the hospital for her mother's belongings. Her main concern was seeing Kathy settled into her next location, which would allow her to feel more comfortable. However, Sarah came across some communication discrepancies with the assisted living facility and after only four months moved her mom to a different location. Because Kathy was in an actual home, she could have a little garden, which she loved. That freedom gave her a sense of independence. The new arrangement also allowed Kathy to explore her wish list.

"When my mom was in the hospital, she wrote a list of things that she wanted to do when she got out. On the top of her list was that she wanted to hug a cow."

Sarah laughed at the bizarreness of her mother's top request. However, who was Sarah to stop Kathy's dreams from coming true?

"So, I took her to a creamery up in Frederick. We went, and fed the baby calves. We had little milk jugs to feed the calves. I have some pictures of her doing that!"

Sarah recalled the look of pure happiness on her mom's face when she was with the cows—at that moment, time had stopped. Life stood still for both Kathy and Sarah. In the sadness of dementia, Sarah was able to hold a moment still and keep the smile on her mom's face present throughout the day. Being realistic, Sarah knew that moment would eventually fade. Soon, Kathy would be back in the living facility to manage her illnesses. During our interview, a few months after hugging the cows, Sarah had another tough decision for Kathy—hospice. Hospice is a mix of emotions for care partners and their loved ones. Often viewed negatively, hospice is intended to be a transition from medical care focused on curing to medical care focused on comfort. Anyone with approximately six months left in life can qualify, and yet most people only use hospice in their last week of life.

"Literally two weeks ago, my mom was so bad that when I was talking to her neurologist on the phone, I was asking, 'Should I consider hospice at this point?' It got that bad."

Phone in hand, Sarah decided to give Kathy more time instead.

Even though Sarah was buying time away from hospice, Kathy's health continued to decline. Although Sarah couldn't fix her mom's condition, she didn't want to count Kathy out before she had the best chance to fight forward. After all, Sarah knew the next move for Kathy would be her last.

"There's moments where I can just see pure joy. When I was taking her to see the cows, I would call her every day and tell her, She would forget, but the day I took her she was so excited. There are moments where it's hard knowing that she'll forget certain things, but when it is a happy moment, it's like a real happy moment because it's like the first time she's hearing it."

During my interview, Kathy was holding on the best way possible. She may not have remembered Sarah when she saw her, but Sarah remembers moments with Kathy. Sarah still keeps Kathy's bucket list with her for motivation. Although the list is incomplete, Sarah promised her mom they would continue to check each item off no matter how long it takes.

I spoke with Sarah for nearly an hour our first time discussing life with her mom. She exposed so much of herself and the painful retold journey with her mom. I felt I may have exhausted her emotionally. She smiled and said she was happy to talk to people about her mom. "It's life," she said. Understanding that life has been difficult for Sarah at such a young age, I felt her stance on optimism would be something other young people can hold onto during their difficult times. Her vision towards optimism is also a reminder of how she was able to fight out of the darkness to bring others into the light.

Sarah wasn't lost for words on the topic of optimism. "I look at optimism day by day. I try to take everything as a learning experience and try to get something out of it. Being in the psychology field, I want to help people. I want to be a counselor."

Sarah's willingness to discuss her struggles from a real-world perspective gives her a greater connection with others she works with in her career as she becomes a therapist. She also sees the support reflecting onto herself. "It will help me in the future for clients with dementia."

38 Days After Our Interview

On December 7, 2023, I received a text that Kathy was in the hospital and would likely pass by the end of the day. Early the next morning, with Sarah by her side, Katherine Allison Close's body gave way to complications from pneumonia.

She was sixty-one. Sarah was twenty-five.

CHAPTER TEN

Debbie and Shannon

THE HOUSE THAT SHANNON BUILT

66 I don't know how much optimism I felt." That was the first thing Shannon said when discussing her life as a care partner for her mother, Debbie. Although many people I spoke with said something similar to Shannon, it wasn't the response I was expecting from a founding member and current President of the YES group. Still, Shannon is not alone in her feelings of negativity towards the idea of optimism when dealing with dementia, let alone when reflecting on how the disease altered their lives. However, she wanted me to recognize off the bat that her story is anything but glamorous.

"It was really heavy. It's hard for me to find the positives in that situation. I was against everybody—against the world. I mean, it just did not seem like this is what I needed to be doing at that point in my life."

No one who finds themselves caring for their parents at an early age imagines it as an obvious step in life. No one is ready regardless of when that time comes. The severity of Debbie's condition completely altered Shannon's way of life.

When Debbie was diagnosed, Shannon was advancing swiftly in the legal profession and married with a husband and two children. Managing a thriving career while trying to be an on-call parent is anything but carefree. Adding Debbie's care to the mix wholly altered every aspect of Shannon's life.

Continuing with her disclaimer about optimism, Shannon said, "I feel like I have a slightly different voice from other care partners." She continued, "I had a very strained relationship with my mom."

As the oldest of five children, Shannon enjoyed the perks of being the only girl among four rowdy boys. As a result, her parents treated Shannon like a princess.

"We used to be as close as a mother and daughter could be, closer than most of my friends were with their parents. I had my own room and my own clothes and I never used to share a bunk bed with my brothers."

Even though her parents were far from wealthy, Shannon's mother portrayed an elevated appearance to the public. Now, as a parent herself, Shannon admits she understood her mother's rationale for wanting people to think everything behind the curtain is impeccable—to a degree. Regardless of how durable a facade may be, it can never stay immaculate forever. Still, her mother dressed all the kids nicely and always made a point to carry herself with tremendous distinction. Shannon said her mother was always impeccably dressed and known for her beauty. Shannon became accustomed to people commenting on how stunning her mother was.

Shannon and her mother remained close until her late teenage years, when, as teenagers do, Shannon began to rebel against the system. "You start to not go along with everything your parents want you to do. That little bit of that separation period, the rebellion period, I feel like we never made a smooth transition into a mother-daughter relationship once I became a young adult."

Their bond became more elastic as Shannon fought for her independence until, finally, their connection had been stretched too far to find its way back to their beginning. "I felt like this person who had been my best friend was more disconnected from me. Maybe because she was still trying to parent me as a young child and not as a young adult. I wasn't having it."

The rift between Shannon and her mother grew wider as Shannon went to college and law school. Shannon found her passion through the law and dove headfirst into a successful career. Even though their personalities changed over time, Shannon would still see her mom in Debbie's role as a high-profile assistant for a judge. Although Shannon doesn't practice the type of law that takes her to court regularly, the times she would have to be in court were always a chance to reconnect with her mom. Debbie would pop her head into a conference room in the court when Shannon would have a meeting just to say hello, and Shannon would do the same. During a visit to her mom's office, Shannon first noticed something wasn't right with Debbie.

"I remember this one day vividly. When I stopped by her work, she wore leggings and a kind of sloppy sweater. She had no makeup on either, and I thought, 'What happened this morning?'"

Seeing Debbie disheveled was entirely out of the norm for someone always known for their refinement, especially at work. Shannon mentioned something to Debbie, but she played it off as being in a rush or too busy, and it wasn't that big of a deal. However, the woman that Shannon had known her whole life would never allow her appearance to take a backseat to being late. Over time, Debbie's unfamiliar appearance became more prevalent.

"She was fifty-seven when I started to notice. By the time dementia affected her performance at work and her ability to function at home, I think she was around fifty-nine."

Shannon spoke up a little louder, and Debbie ignored the signs again. She was never a big believer in therapy or bettering one's mental health. After several attempts from Shannon, Debbie begrudgingly gave in to seeing someone. Neither of them knew what to expect when contacting medical professionals. Shannon shrugged her shoulders when thinking back to that appointment. "I took her to a general psychiatrist. They diagnosed her with Generalized Anxiety Disorder and Major Depressive Disorder." Adding an exhale of frustration from that day, Shannon said, "Then, they send us on our way with the normal litany of medications for those disorders."

Shannon was convinced there was more to her mom's condition than a few pills could cure. However, in classic Debbie fashion, she deflected Shannon's views of her behavior as nonsense. "It was so funny. There she was again, trying to put on, telling the doctor this is an appointment for me. I'm just sitting there letting her say her thing as she's painting this perfect picture."

The doctor couldn't tell, but that appointment ended Debbie's plastic facade. Finally, Shannon had heard enough.

"I said to the doctor, 'Am I allowed to interject? Do you want to know what I have to say?' Then, I spilled the beans. Still, the doctor didn't see anything more than depression and anxiety."

From the brief time I've known Shannon, I can picture her lawyer side growing agitated by the doctor's ignorance and Debbie's ability to play him. Not that depression and anxiety are anything to gloss over, but Shannon knew in her heart that the evidence was pointing to something else more severe. She would end up being right. Sadly, it took another two and a half to three years after that initial doctor visit to get an accurate diagnosis of Debbie's condition: Lewy Body Dementia (LBD).

A natural researcher, Shannon absorbed as much medical content as she could about her mother's condition. Once she started reading documents about the disease, there was no denying that Debbie had been suffering for quite some time. "Once you see it in black and white," Shannon said, "it describes the behaviors we knew for sure, and the testing confirmed it."

"What did your siblings say about that?"

Shannon gave a "big sister knows best" smile. "I'm task oriented. It's not like we had a family meeting, and we all cried and held hands," Shannon said, knowing she would be the one to take charge. "It's like, 'I'm sending links to academic journals, here's the diagrams, it starts in this part of the brain, then it progresses here and so forth.' Now you have it."

I envision her laying out the rules for Debbie's welfare as if briefing her team for a big case. Shannon continued discussing the materials she provided her siblings, outlining where they all stood. "I was trying to be on top of it. I was controlling it."

"Is anybody else in the family a lawyer?"

"No. Just me."

"Because it's a very lawyerly way of talking about it," I said while laughing out of respect for her aggressive approach to Debbie.

Thankfully, Shannon appreciated my observation and agreed. "It's the way my brain works. That's what law school does to you. It brainwashes everything you knew before and teachers you only to think this one way, and I felt that was an effective way. It worked well because my brothers were the counterbalance to that."

Shannon focused on making sure the medications were filled, the appointments were scheduled, and that Debbie did everything she was supposed to do. Her brothers' mentality went more on the emotional side of the disease. Shannon didn't have time for that. Relying on emotional support is just one part of being a care partner. Not only does it take a village to care for someone with dementia, but with Lewy Body Dementia, the immediate and eventual care goes far beyond simply being an emotional shoulder to lean on. Shannon's approach towards Debbie's care was completely built around love and comfort for her mother. To provide that, you have to have a plan.

Although Shannon's legal education strengthened her mind around ensuring all goals were met on time, it also prepared her for handling when the strategy went sideways. Shannon knew that Debbie's independence would be fractured and eventually eliminated by the effects of Lewy Body. Despite this, Shannon wanted to allow her mother to live alone despite her reservations.

"This began to add stress to our relationship because she felt like now I'm pushing her into these different places to live."

Although Shannon's motives for finding Debbie a proper living facility were genuine, if not determined, Shannon also knew it would be a good experiment. Shannon wanted Debbie to remain secure and independent. Alternatively, Debbie's inability to do so would show how incapable she was anywhere other than a setting that offered assistance. Shannon combed the area for several options that would best meet Debbie's needs; however, something else was still missing. Continuing to come up empty, Shannon realized there was one more place to consider.

Shannon and her husband have worked very hard in their careers, and their beautiful home is a sign of that. They realized there was room for more than the four of them.

"My had dad moved in with us when we bought this house. Not because he needed care but because the arrangement worked well."

Shannon's parents divorced after she finished high school, and she and her father remained as close as any father and daughter could be. She always looked to him for guidance and support, but the transition was never easy, despite his support for her. When he moved in, there was no plan to add Debbie eventually. For starters, she was still able to live on her own. Secondly, what child would ever want their elderly divorced parents to cohabitate after decades of divorce? As a child of divorce myself, even if I lived in a twenty-room mansion with a moat and drawbridge dividing a palatial estate, I can't imagine doing that for them. I was intrigued.

"He had a very strange relationship with my mom, but we knew there was no choice but to move her in. He lived on the main floor, and she lived right below us. They each had their living quarters right above and below each other."

"That had to have been interesting," I teased.

"I could get a TV show deal for sure," she replied.

"I understand all interactions after divorce are tricky, but he was watching his ex-wife. I imagined that was unique?"

"I think it was hard for him," she said. "He developed another level of compassion for her. He would tolerate her a little bit more than he did previously. I do think it was a lot for him to watch what was happening. And to be candid with you, I think my dad never really stopped loving my mom."

Her father's dedication to both her and her mother was a testament to the culture Shanon created in her home. She could have looked at the situation and thought the dividing wall should be the only answer. Still, Shannon wanted to bridge the gap between her young but aging parents, who were also nurtured by her two children, whom she calls old souls. When Debbie moved into Shannon's home in 2017, her son was nine, and her daughter was six. The kids were hardly of the age to understand the dynamic of divorce, elder care, or Lewy Body Dementia, let alone Young-Onset Dementia. However, despite their youth, Shannon said her kids were mature enough to handle the severity of the situation.

"How was that relationship with seeing their grandmother?"

Shannon's face brightens every time she talks about her children. She can't commend her children enough for their patience and poise. "My kids, they're just," she began, trying to find the best words to describe them, "...they're just wise," she said.

Handling the level of emotional intelligence it takes to hold one, let alone two, aging grandparents living in your house takes more than wisdom. When Shannon told me more about her kid's approach to their living situation, it was clear they were gifted with an incredible sense of grace. In a nature versus nurture observation, her children witnessed Shannon's compassion for her mom, teaching them the length of support family provides for one another.

"They were never the types of kids you interact with as little kids. We always talk to them as adults. They knew the situation was weird. I would try to say the strange behavior doesn't matter because this is your grandmother. But I mean, she would annoy the hell out of them, and they didn't want to deal with it. I would try to strike a balance between how much you force your kids to try to spend time with their grandparents while letting them have their own space when they need it."

I relayed my story about seeing my Bubbe in the same state and around the same age as her kids. "I would hear her say certain things that were off. Then, she would start with outbursts, and then she went to the nursing home."

Shannon nodded in agreement.

"To your credit, like my dad did, I always think about the fact that he would take me to see her, regardless of her condition. It was like, you have to understand what's going on. It was sometimes quick visits, but not always. Still, it's hard for kids to understand, especially at that age."

The concept of children understanding the world of dementia is another reason I wanted to share the Optimistics story. There are going to be children like Shannon's who can open their minds and emote how they're feeling, while others will turn away to disregard the disease without wanting to understand it. For care partners like Shannon, there is a duty to bring the realities of dementia into the light rather than keep it tucked away like an antique no one notices.

"I think it also draws attention again to the different types of dementia," Shannon said. "I'm not in any way suggesting that everybody with dementia is pleasantly confused. Some people are very passive and pleasantly confused, and they're kind of easy to be around. But there was a constant fluctuation in my mom's cognitive function."

Debbie's mood swings and ability to self-reason were aspects of her condition that could not be ignored and had a tremendous impact on the entire household.

"Some days were good, some days were really bad. The behaviors and the aggression, and the hallucinations—auditory hallucinations, visual hallucinations—the crazy and the emotional outbursts and that type of thing are traumatic."

Actions like that made Shannon's kids even more concerned about the severity of Debbie's condition than they initially could comprehend. "This leaves your kids wondering, 'What is Grandma seeing?'"

Shannon took a pause. I sensed she was back in one of those moments.

"It was traumatic," she said softly.

Shannon did her best to work with Debbie's outbursts, but sometimes the animosity was too much to contain.

"It disrupted our lives. On a Halloween occasion, she was completely off the deep end. My husband, my kids, and I were going to go to our neighbors together, but I was in some sort of a hostage negotiation situation with my mom to let me go. It was that type of behavior and outburst that I constantly observed that made trying to both be a mom to my kids and then a mom to my mom, was really different."

I spoke to Shannon about the similar sense of role reversal that I've seen in other care partners. Children become parents to their parents and spouses become personal nurses. This is a part of life that people foresee happening down the road and not at an age when there is still so much more life left to live.

"Was she understanding what was going on? Did she understand that you brought her to your house to care for her?"

Shannon shook her head. "No. It was all painted in a negative light. She understood it, but to her, it was like her jail cell. It was a hundred-thousand-dollar apartment that we built! I mean it literally could be like in a senior living magazine," she added.

I found this next part of Shannon's story incredibly endearing, unlike anyone else I interviewed. Every care partner living with someone alters their living conditions to help their loved one. This could be adding more railings, adjusting the structures of bathrooms, or even updating technology in the home. Never one for the status quo, Shannon isn't one to simply follow the normal trends. Shannon did her research... and then some.

Her voice rose with a bolt of energy. "I downloaded software for the specifics of a living facility. No transitions on the floors and the $5,000 tiny little roll-in accessible shower thing with rubber. Everything! I added a washer and dryer, a full kitchen, all the things! I redid my driveway so she wouldn't have to pass through my house to get to her house."

I was in awe. "That's incredible!"

Shannon spoke faster. "I wanted to do everything I could do to make her feel like she was on her own, and as if I was just there to support her. But she felt like she was just locked in the basement. That's what she would tell a stranger."

All I could offer was shaking my head.

Shannon breathed, saying, "Yeah, that was fun for me."

We both laughed out of relief.

"Even after you spent all this money and made a nice, beautiful place," I said, still laughing.

Shannon rolled her eyes. "Yup, we just threw her in the basement," she said sarcastically.

Using what little resources her mother had available to build a state-of-the-art addition to her house, Shannon knew money wouldn't be the ultimate answer. Although she wasn't expecting weekly handwritten letters of affirmation from Debbie, Shannon was crushed by her mom's lack of positive expressions of gratitude. When Shannon would step back to look at the life of comfort and security she created for Debbie, only to be treated with disdain, it added to the reasons Shannon told me from the start: why she lacks optimism.

"Shannon, it's beyond impressive what you did, but again, you're not the first person I spoke to who isn't happy-go-lucky about this. Especially with Lewy Body, so I commend you for it."

My compliments to Shannon aren't anything new to her, and I'm glad to hear that. I believe there isn't a single person alive who doesn't look at what Shannon's family did to improve Debbie's life without the utmost admiration. Even if she didn't see it the same way, Shannon was preparing for the next stage of Debbie's care, when having a soft bed and people around are the last memories they will have together.

"She was with you for three and a half years. Did she ever have to go somewhere else, or did she pass away at the house?

"No. Ultimately, she passed at the house."

"I'm sorry," I offered.

"Earlier, when she had moved in, the doctor we went to see was part of this outpatient clinic at a very beautiful memory care facility near my house. It would have been ideal."

Shannon thought back to when she would take Debbie to that clinic for appointments and laughed at Debbie's positive response. "When we'd go there, she would always call it beautiful," she said, thrilled at a plausible option.

"I knew she didn't want to go there. I told her, 'I can schedule when I help you shower. I can schedule your meals. I can schedule when I clean your room. I can schedule when we go to the doctor, but I can't schedule when you need to use the bathroom.'"

Bathroom hygiene issues are a constant concern of care partners. It's uncomfortable to address and to handle physically and causes the most stress for care partners. One care partner told me that she could handle everything to a degree, but when her husband began to lose the ability to control his bowels, she realized she had reached her limit. It's not only the hygienic aspect of the bathroom. It's the lack of control a person with dementia has over their own body that is the means for the most concern if not the care partner's final breaking point. Shannon did all she could, but her life was not at the point where she could babysit Debbie at that level.

"I can't not work. I have to work. I run the law firm! I have my kids." She said, as if defending her case, even though no one could disagree with her work in making Debbie feel safe.

Shannon said that she explored the options of moving her mom to a place that would provide the hygienic assistance she needed. Still, at that point, Debbie's disorientation of her surroundings became too intense to handle another move. Debbie already looked at Shannon's immaculate home as a prison, and anything new would likely cause more trouble than relief. Over the years, there were medical instances where Debbie had to be admitted overnight. She would become delirious while in the hospital, which is common for people with dementia. This can make their cognitive status even worse and cause more delusions or hallucinations.

"It became more challenging for me when she was not here due to her level of hysteria because she still had her cell phone. She would call me and you would have thought she was being murdered in the hospital," Shannon said with an exhausted memory. She added, "That was more traumatic for me than just keeping her here and dealing with the trouble."

Unwilling to be in a hospital, the level of home care attention comes with a hefty price. Debbie had almost no money left for such treatment, so Shannon once again reached into her own pockets for her mother's care. The cost of in-home treatment is jarring. I prefer the term criminal. I'm not diminishing the professionalism of any care provider or the quality of service offered, but I can't help feeling that the industry is built on the nature of debilitating circumstances. Guilt and limited options have become the supply and demand of the home nursing industry. Just ask Shannon.

"It's the toughest position because you feel morally obligated, but you will impoverish yourself." Shannon added, "I spent her last twenty grand for two weeks!"

I thought I misheard her.

"That can't be! Two weeks?"

"Yeah, two weeks."

To make matters worse, Shannon was not getting any relief now that she hired help. It meant she took on extra roles of coordinator, supervisor, and trainer of the caregivers.

"I was the new Care Coordinator. I was the Supervisor of the Caregivers who I had to reorient and go downstairs for training every twelve hours."

The mental and now physical agony Shannon was putting herself through daily for Debbie started to reach her "apex of unmanageability," as she described it. After counseling with others having gone through this, the topic of hospice was raised as a possible next step for Debbie. The word hospice took over Shannon's consciousness like a virus. She knew what hospice meant, and no one came back from it. Even if it's for several months at best, Shannon had difficulty accepting the next level of care for Debbie. After several rounds of research, Shannon found a service that brought hospice to her home, which would make Debbie the most comfortable in her final days.

"It escalated so sharply and so quickly," Shannon said softly when talking about the process of hospice. "We were all breaking down."

Shannon looked away. Then said, "And then that was the end."

Shannon had a priest come into their home and give Debbie her last rites. Her brothers also joined her at the house, taking turns sitting with Debbie. Not only did this allow Shannon and her siblings to take a mental health break from the inevitable, but the alone time gave everyone a chance to have a private conversation with Debbie. Shannon had several conversations with her mom over the years, conjuring up a new set of emotions between mother and daughter.

"Were you able to make peace with everything? Especially about your relationship with her at the end."

Shannon's answer wasn't what I expected.

"No. To be honest with you, no, I don't think that I made peace with it. I do think that I was able to set aside my issues long enough to truly feel the loss of my mom."

For the first time during our talk, Shannon's stern take on dementia began to lower as she thought about Debbie's final days.

"Ugh, you're going to trigger me, Richie," she said with a quiver in her lip and a wink of humor.

"Don't worry about that," I said, trying to play off any discomfort she may have been feeling. I smiled and told her, "It's okay. Everybody cries when I talk to them."

"No, it's fine. It's good. These are the things that I box away. I think I was able to suppress my feelings long enough to tell her that I loved her."

Shannon's eyes watered. "I felt at that moment I had just lost my mom. Also to feel the moment of 'now we're orphans.' I was, at the time, thirty-nine years old, and I was an adult orphan. That's weird to me. All of my friends' parents are still here, and now, mine are all gone."

This was the first time I realized how young Shannon was when Debbie died. In addition, in the years before that, as a young woman, she had to alter her life to support her mother. It had taken a toll on Shannon, but she would never have done it differently. The night of Debbie's passing, Shannon and her brothers went into her backyard and all sat together, absorbing the realities of their new lives without their mother. They sat silently for a while, but soon, the tension was broken, thanks to her brother Kevin.

Disrupting the somber moment with her siblings, Kevin said, "Guys, if our parents are gone, then we can do whatever we want!"

The gentle release of tension between them was exactly what they needed. Shannon said, "You idiot, we're all married, we've got kids. We've been doing what we want for a long time now."

Shannon's smile while talking about her brothers is a refreshing addition to Debbie's passing. She said, "It was kind of perfect. We just acknowledged losing a second parent in a very short amount of time, and it also just kind of brought us together in this moment of inappropriate youth."

Returning to Shannon's original idea of optimism, she added one addendum.

"The financial doom and gloom that accompanies this process, the optimistic spin is that there are strategies and options. The most overwhelming and least optimistic you could feel is just going based on what your friends have told you or going based on what you can find on the internet. There's too much misinformation, and you could be missing opportunities."

I found Shannon's story had a rather unconventional take on optimism as someone who lives life based on fact over faith. Shannon's tale is more about hope than she may realize. There is no sugarcoating Debbie's condition (it was one of the worst I encountered). The lessons were unlike any others I met along this journey. Shannon could have shut down and closed the door on Debbie, given their trying relationship. Instead, she guided her mom the entire way. Shannon could have asked her four siblings to take turns and have Debbie serve her final months in a carousel of homes with no sense of security. But she rebuilt her life and house for Debbie. Shannon could have remained one-dimensional in her mother's dealings; however, she refused to do anything but stay present, even if her mom didn't have the capacity to appreciate it.

Shannon's life is also a lesson in what it means to serve a community that desperately needs guidance and has long been ignored. Today, Shannon uses her legal skills to focus on helping individuals find the best solutions for care partners and family members in her position. Debbie would be proud of the work her daughter does for others.

Shannon has devoted her professional life to supporting her clients' needs and has become a champion for dementia and Alzheimer's through her philanthropy. As one of the twelve 2024 Alzheimer's Association Memory Ball Dancing Stars, Shannon has been training for months and beating the ground for donations. Not surprisingly, as I write this, Shannon leads the other dancers by over twenty thousand dollars and shows no sign of stopping until she breaks the record. I'd expect nothing less from her.

On Shannon's donation page, she writes:

"I'm dancing FOR MY MOM because it reminds me of the 13 years of my childhood I spent dancing—my mom was my biggest cheerleader—before her life was taken away decades too soon.

—I'm dancing to raise AWARENESS OF YOUNG-ONSET DEMENTIA!

—I'm dancing to support research to END ALL FORMS OF DEMENTIA!

—I'm dancing to SUPPORT SANDWICH GENERATION CARE PARTNERS!"

At the time of this writing the official tally has not been calculated to demonstrate Shannon's incredible work for the Memory Ball, but Shannon has already won. She's made it past the darkest demons of dementia, fought off the isolation Lewy Body Dementia brings, and gracefully handled the unrelenting pressure of watching a parent deteriorate in front of your eyes.

On December 6, 2020, exactly six months after her sixty-sixth birthday, Debbie took her final breath. She was surrounded by the love of her children and grandchildren in the comfort of a home built precisely for this very moment.

CHAPTER ELEVEN

Donna and Alisha

X-IT TO EXIT

"She was like me...She was living two lives."

Every Optimistic knows the line your mind crosses when you get your official diagnosis, but it's never as defined for their families. This isn't about acceptance of having dementia—that you can't argue with—but it's how it affects the people around the diagnosis that takes many shapes. Alisha can't recall at what age she learned her mother had dementia because she was never told when it started. What Alisha *can* recall is being a young teen and having a mother who seemed to defy everything Alisha wanted to do.

"I was in sixth grade but I remember we had to write in our journal every day for language arts. I wrote about how my mom and I were fighting every day. I was going to school in tears on the bus every single day. I wrote in my journal how I don't know who this woman is anymore—but she's not my mom. I didn't know where she'd gone."

Alisha's teacher confronted her about her journaling but Alisha was unable to make her teacher understand and rightfully so; Alisha didn't either. On the surface, Alisha's rebellious views towards her mother were chalked up to being teen angst or mother-daughter scuffles over childish disputes that usually get settled over ice cream, but there was much more. Donna was acting completely out of character; no longer nurturing or compassionate, with massive mood swings, and making up stories that weren't true. Even though Alisha would argue the contrary, it's hard to believe a teen over their parents, let alone when they are already acting out in their own right. This further divided Alisha and her mom. The rift between them caused by their mutual misunderstanding increased over the next few years. Alisha's once pristine image of her mother twisted into that of a disgruntled stranger.

Before adopting Alisha, Donna obtained a doctorate in molecular biology and worked as a Marine Scientist. She later became one of the first Physician's Assistants in the country as the field developed in the late sixties. Donna was bright and philanthropic, volunteering for various charities and donating to animal causes. Even when she left the field to raise Alisha and her brother, Donna was on the board of the local zoo. She would bring wild animals into their school to show the students. Donna would also lead science lessons at their school as well.

"She was such an attentive parent. She signed us up for every sport that we could do and then helped us pick the one that we were best at. She wasn't a mom who just dropped us off and picked us up."

Donna was the poster parent for all things right when it came to showing Alisha how a mother should act. Donna was at all their school events, on the sidelines, and cheering Alisha on, regardless of how well she did. When Alisha was bullied for being one of the only Asian kids in a predominantly white community, Donna comforted her. Donna was the first one with a bandage when Alisha fell off her bike and knew what to say to make her forget about the fall. Donna would playfully point out if there were a cute boy, knowing it would make Alisha blush. Over time, Donna became Alisha's sounding board for dating advice.

"I had social anxiety at events or birthday parties or whatever it was. She was so happy to hold my hand or be right next to me or right behind me. She was my rock in so many ways."

Alisha was always proud of how her mom attracted people around her and enamored by how impressed others were with her accomplishments. When looking at her mother in such high regard as an intellect, Alisha would never have thought that her mom's brain would ever be an issue. So, when Donna's mood swings became more constant, Alisha internalized that anger as something she did. When Donna lost her patience with others such as friends, people in public, and even Alisha's father, it only confirmed her altered views of Donna. Not only did Alisha stop trusting her mother's intuition, but Donna also stopped trusting herself. In turn, it aided in her inability to connect with Alisha like she had in the past.

Her erratic behavior became a constant nuisance to Alisha. The smallest task would aggravate Donna and Alisha would bear the brunt of her mom's inability to accept help.

"Teaching her how to open an email, or exit out of the email, or how to get to the email," Alisha told me while pointing at the keyboard, still in frustration. "I'm like, 'Mom, you just have to press the giant X. An X means to exit, you know? You X-it to exit.' I thought it was so simple!" Donna would confirm the directions, only to need help again moments later.

"She's like, 'X-it to exit, got it,' then, five minutes later she would say, 'Wait, Alicia, how do I get out of this?'. Oh, my gosh, Mom! Then it's how to turn on the TV, how to navigate our universal TV remote, which no one can even do anyways."

Donna's inability to do automatic tasks that most toddlers can handle continued to push Alisha to various breaking points of teenage brashness. Everything Donna did bothered Alisha. Ironically, both of them couldn't understand why this was happening.

"I remember when my dad first sat me down because Mom and I were getting into fights and screaming at each other. And I would say things like, 'Are you crazy or something?' because he wasn't taking my side. Then, he would say, 'I need you to never say that again because your mom just got a diagnosis that we're gonna look into further'"

The diagnosis stage of dementia is the line that splits your world in two; wondering what is wrong and confirming what is fact. It didn't make sense to Alisha at first, "My mom? She's so bright, successful, respected. *My* mom?" Then, after the diagnosis—and the new world begins—it did. Before, as Mike once mentioned, "Alzheimer's doesn't care what you've accomplished."

While Donna's life began on a new path of acceptance of her reality, Alisha went deep into a world of substance abuse to dim her reality. Those with substance abuse disorders will tell you that there are their drug friends and their clean friends; each plays a key part in numbing whatever pain your body is battling. Alisha modeled her parents' academic success inside the classroom with clean friends who looked at her as someone with a wide-open future. Those friends had no idea of Alisha's other life in dimly lit places, with cocktails of anything she could find to silence her pain.

"I started partying. It didn't help that I was this Asian nerd in a sea of white people in Oklahoma. I wanted to do everything to fit in. And I just wanted to be cool."

Alisha hid both social groups from one another in fear that combining the two would destroy one of them. However, as a frustrated teenager watching her home life flip on its head, she wasn't sure which she wanted to lose. Eventually, the choice wasn't her own and drugs became her only confidant.

Alisha rolled her eyes with a sheepish grin. "I don't know if this is appropriate for your book," she said with a slight blush.

I smiled back. "It's fine. Please."

Alisha leaned forward in her seat and laughed before she even talked.

"I was fifteen or something, and I had to take care of my mom at the house and I started smoking weed. And, the first time that I got high, I was watching my mom while my dad had to take an overnight shift at the hospital."

We both laughed and as someone who would have been considered her nerdy friend if we grew up together, I can't even imagine what teenage Alisha was thinking.

"But, it was the first time that I had a good time with my mom in many years."

"Because you're high?"

"I was high. She had short-term memory loss and I had short-term memory loss. And we were just laughing at the same mistakes that both of us would make. She would start saying something and stop and we would start laughing. You know, at this point, my mom has no filter. She called me out on things I was doing; like I was laying in bed and I guess I was breathing loudly."

Alisha looks off to the side, smiling while she recalls the exact moments she could hide with laughter. "She was like, 'Hey, stop doing that!' and I didn't even realize I was doing it. So I started laughing then she started laughing. She was also at that point where she probably didn't even know why she was laughing. It was the fact that I was in a light mood for the first time in so many years and she was in a light mood. I felt my empathy for her situation expanded tremendously. I realized, 'Oh my gosh, like what she must be going through,' you know? I should not be getting mad at her for not being able to turn on the TV anymore. Certain things like that."

Alisha bonded with Donna for a short time on an unconventional level. As beautiful as that experience was, it was also a gateway to other things. The pain Alisha hid outweighed any minimal joyous moments Donna could provide. The insecurities drugs could hide became more important and Alisha began experimenting with various substances. Ultimately, drinking consumed her life.

"I didn't have any support. I didn't know where to go. And I think part of why I got into that, I don't want to call it a community, but the wrong group. We were all troubled kids with broken families who are all trying to cope and self-medicate our depression."

Alisha's growing anxiety convinced her that leaving the house would be the best for her mom. Maybe space and time away from her mom would help to reattach their divided bond. Alisha used college as the best excuse to hide Donna's dementia and having to cope with knowing she would soon lose her mom. While other friends her age looked at their parents as embarrassing by being quirky and joking around with friends, Alisha hid Donna from those close to her.

"To be completely honest my friends had absolutely no idea how to react because I don't think any of them truly understood what Alzheimer's is. I think it made it a little awkward when they would come to my house because they didn't know how to talk to my mom. They just kind of acted almost like she wasn't there."

Looking back today, Alisha knows the person who was too ashamed of her mother is not the same mature adult now, but that realization can't change the past. The same idea is shared by many children of people with dementia who believe looking away from themselves will allow others not to see the truth. For Alisha, who had feet in two different worlds, keeping Donna's condition hidden only caused her depression to become more exposed at the surface.

"I had my dark secret side; partying on the weekends and sneaking out of the house and doing drugs," she said, "And when my nerd friends— and I hate the sound of calling them that, but that's what we were—found out, they were so upset with me. And that's when I realized that they really didn't understand because I'm like, 'You saw my mom's condition. How can you be mad that I'm going out and just trying to have some fun,' you know?"

As a person with a substance and alcohol use disorder, Alisha was projecting onto others to rationalize her decisions. This further pushed away her stable friends, leading her into the accepting arms of her substance use disorder. While Alisha continued to fall deeper into areas that eased her pain, the rock that was Donna for her when she was younger, became a boulder that could no longer be tucked away. Still, Alisha tried.

Ironically, the isolation that Alisha was experiencing was similar to Donna's condition. Isolation is one of the hardest aspects of Alzheimer's. Regardless if you have several family and friends around you, or the highest level of care money can buy, being isolated is a mental state, not a physical one. Drugs can make the pain subside, and long walks with a loved one holding your hand can give you compassion, but your brain controls how you view isolation. Eventually, when Alisha was a sophomore in college, Donna's mind consumed her body, and there was no other choice but to move her to hospice. She survived for almost half a year there, but it was clear from day one Donna would never return home.

"By the time she was in hospice, she couldn't walk anymore, she had to be fed. She lost a lot of weight. And the final, day, she was basically on life support."

While home for the holidays, Alisha's dad told her Donna's time had run out. "She was on a lot of pain medications, so she wasn't in any pain—but we needed to make a decision."

Donna had become a shell with only tubes and devices helping her to breathe. Seeing his wife in such an extreme state, he told his children that he didn't want them to see their mom when she took her final breath, which he knew was imminent. For years, he had prepared himself for this exact moment, and as a physician, he had seen hundreds of people pass. None that he loved as much as Donna. In her solitude, he was support, and knowing how death can change families, this was a moment just for the two of them. When Alisha's father called her two days later to tell her Donna had passed away peacefully, for the first time Alisha can recall, he choked up.

Even though Alisha couldn't be there for the final moment of Donna's life, she had her moment with Donna beforehand. Alisha sat with her mother, knowing Donna could not understand her. Alisha wanted her mom to hear that Alisha was doing well, yet that was a lie.

"I remember telling her, like, 'You know, I'm doing good, Mom. I'm in school like you should be. I just want you to be proud,' even though I was doing terribly. I actually wasn't okay. I was trying to stay sober, trying to do well in school but frankly, I was flunking out. I was so depressed. I just wanted to do drugs and I couldn't. I think I was probably drinking at the time. I wanted to focus on her more because, in my life, everything wasn't going okay."

Everyone I've interviewed looked at their final conversation with their loved one as the finish line to a marathon they had been running for years. Some conversations are filled with guilt, and some are apologetic. Others talk about love, God, and finally being free. Regardless, they just want them to know their lives will continue in their honor. Alisha wasn't truthful with her mom, but can you blame her?

"There's only so many options I feel like that we have in those moments, you know?"

"It was beautiful," I told her. "I would have done the same thing."

I asked Alisha how she viewed optimism. In the face of her mother's passing and knowing what she has been through, what is her take on life that should be etched in stone?

"Being optimistic is a secret weapon. Going forward positively is to accept that reality is not idea. Being able to allow yourself to feel everything that you feel, even when it's not positive, is the best route to staying optimistic. It's a secret weapon against all the darkness that surrounds us. I think that's what people don't understand, is that if you don't feel it, if you reject it, if you try to push it away, then you stay stuck."

I nodded as Alisha continued and couldn't help but feel that the words she was saying to me were ones she wished her mother could understand now.

"If you allow yourself to feel it and feel sad and just let it happen and you stop fighting it, that's where you feel more at peace. And then when you're at peace, you're able to help everyone around you better and you're able to honor the person that you're caring for or that you have cared for."

Alisha paused and then revealed something else she hadn't told me yet. "I've gone through substance use and alcohol use disorders, and I even got cancer at one point. I went through chemo and radiation and I did it alone while my family was in Oklahoma. What's insane though, is they always tell you while you're in it, like, this is just making you stronger."

Alisha took a moment to dry her eyes, then said, "Then you're just like, 'I don't want to be strong. I just want this to end.'"

When Alisha mentioned the end, I imagined how often she had to face herself in the mirror, tears falling, makeup smeared, and alone, she saw Donna take shape over her face. Although she and Donna don't share the same DNA, a mother and daughter are forever bound by more than bloodlines. They're united by compassion. Sure, they argued but for a longer time, they laughed. They quarreled over teenage drama, but that didn't stop Donna from being there to hold Alisha's hand, even if Alisha wanted to pull away. It didn't take an alcohol use disorder or cancer to make Alisha see the connection she always had with her mother, but it did shape the idea of what being a mother is to Alisha.

"All I've been through is a tiny grain of sand compared to the beach that my mom's illness was in my life. When I think about who my mom was and how I remember her, I remember her for exactly who she was before she got sick. That's a big part of who I am today."

Alisha's life now is starkly different from where she was during Donna's final days. Seven years after her mother's death, Alisha finally got sober and remains so to this day, turning her bedside final words into a stunning reality, and a lie into the truth.

On January 7, 2015, Donna passed away with her husband by her side. She was sixty-four.

CHAPTER TWELVE

Shara and Audra

3 AM DREAMS

Audra has a confident swagger when she talks as if everything is simply chill. In my work, I come across people who fake a calm demeanor, but Audra is about as real as it gets. She talks like an old friend, smiles at your jokes, has tattoos on her arms, and says she's an open book. I learned that her casualness comes from her years on the golf course, playing against hundreds of people who believed they were better than her. She walked past them, eyed the hole, and sank a putt for an eagle. After a while, knowing your competition is surveilling you from the moment you step onto the green, you learn to ignore the childish smirks that seem to say, "This girl isn't on my level."

They're right—she's better.

Many of Audra's fondest memories with her mother, Shara, are on the golf course. Her mother was always there, from driving her to practice and games to cheering her on. Audra was a three-time Female Player of the Year at High Point University. She catapulted to the top of the conference and later became a golf professional, Audra was certified through the LPGA as an LPGA Teaching & Club Professional. All through her competitive playing years and for the start of her career in the industry, Shara was there for the ride. Eventually, Audra left Maryland and settled in Tampa. Honing her craft on courses in the sunshine state, Audra never missed a phone call with Shara.

"My mom and I were like best friends," Audra said with a smirk. "We talked every single day my whole life, until she started showing the symptoms. We'd talk for hours on the phone, whether in college, Florida, or wherever I lived."

Audra thought something was wrong when the conversations began to skip their regular schedule. On one hand, it's just a phone call, and everyone gets busy, even moms. At the same time, Shara and her siblings began to miss more than just phone calls with Audra. At the time, neither of them even thought about bringing that up with each other. However, Audra's sporadic eyebrow raises turned into deep concern when her mom tried to avoid a trip to Florida. A typical trip would be something Shara would talk about constantly, like a child too excited to contain themselves. Plus, Shara loved the water. Nothing could separate her from a cool breeze and the hot sun, especially with her children.

"The first time the symptoms started showing was when she was very reserved and anxious about coming to Florida to see me and didn't want to fly. She was just very timid. That was the biggest first symptom. It wasn't necessarily a time for me that I thought that she was losing memory."

Around that same time, Audra's siblings began to discuss Shara's condition as a family. "I just thought her personality was different. She didn't want to go out for my sister's graduation party in Morgantown, West Virginia. She was very reserved and left early."

Shara's actions didn't add up to the mother they knew or the ex-wife that Audra's father was used to, either. Even though they got divorced when Audra was nine, her mom and dad always communicated. Yet, the night in Morgantown showed something they all were thinking.

When Shara left the weekend social events, Audra's dad told his kids, "That's weird. Your mom would never leave something like that early."

Audra added, "Things like that were troubling at the time."

Concerns about Shara were made official on June 4, 2018, when Shara was diagnosed with Alzheimer's Dementia. She was only fifty-six at the time. Although she had stopped driving a year before, the official line of having something to point to had been drawn that summer. Dementia became an unmovable anchor in the sand, which Audra and her siblings could no longer dismiss as questionable. They had mixed feelings about that day, as any soon-to-be care partner would.

At first, it was reassuring. They could find the proper medication and care to match her needs. On the other hand, the stress of ensuring Shara has the attention she requires became the main topic of conversation between the siblings and Shara's husband, Scott. Audra couldn't help but lean on the negative side of realizing the fear that would come with her mother's future.

—*Scott is a fantastic husband, but is this too much for one person?*

—*How could Audra help from Florida?*

—*What could her siblings do?*

—*Financially, how will this affect everyone's future?*

Once again, questions with no answers played on repeat in their heads.

"When she was diagnosed, how did that affect how she looked at things?"

"She was terrified of everything," Audra said, massaging her forehead. "I think she became very quiet, just as a human being. Not very talkative; very scared to do anything. She really wouldn't go anywhere without my stepdad. She stopped working and everything. She essentially lost her freedom."

After the diagnosis, Shara and Scott came to Florida for a visit. It was overly emotional for Audra because she knew visits like this may be the last of Shara's life. It was also a reminder of Audra's initial thought that she needed to be closer to her mom.

"I remember her sitting on the porch at our condo in Florida, and she stared off into space. I looked at her, and I thought, what was going through her head? Because I'm looking at her," Audra said, taking a breath to calm her nerves, "and my heart was broken."

Audra watched as Shara sat motionless in a trance, both physically and mentally. The summer sun of Florida's heat beat down on Shara's face as she welcomed its comfort. Usually, her mom would be the first to gather the kids for the water whenever summer came around. Shara loved the water. However, she became a blank canvas, waiting for others to tell her where to go and when. Audra leaned against the porch door frame, wiping her tears away. She yearned for the mom she grew up with to grab her hand for the beach and splash in the relief of the calm waters against their overheated bodies. Instead, Audra would be grabbing Shara's hand simply for reassurance—for both of them.

After four months of introspection, Audra moved back to Maryland for good. To this day, Audra never told Shara why she was returning home. Some things, even for best friends like them, are better left unsaid despite being obvious.

"I can't imagine what it would be like knowing that you have this diagnosis and how your life's going to be. I don't know. I mean, I guess it was me looking at her and thinking of the future essentially. You see her, she's still her, you know? She still looks like her normal self because her body hasn't quit on her yet. But something is going on in her head, and I was like…" Then Audra looked away and back at me. "I just, I don't know."

Audra began to trail off again, then told me, "I still catch myself just staring at her, even now."

"What are you thinking about when you see her now?" I asked.

I'm just trying to figure it out. Like, figuring out what is going on with her, even though she doesn't know, but trying to have that connection somehow. I've noticed recently that she's declined quickly in the last couple of months. But if you look at her in her eyes, she will lock your eyes and know who you are. She might not say your name, but it's all about connection, and that was my way of reading the situation.

A key to being an Optimistic is not only connection but keeping that connection for as long as possible. A steady bond between a loved one with dementia and a care partner is essential for the mental health of both parties. With that, it can be challenging for care partners like Audra to keep that connection going when there is no back-and-forth in the communication.

"When you visit her now, how are you talking to her? Does she understand? Is she more reserved and silent?"

Audra is happy to share Shara's current state, knowing her family is on the "fortunate" side of caring for a person with Alzheimer's when it comes to communication.

"Oh yeah, she loves just to talk! About what? Well, I don't even know what she's talking about sometimes. She did call me her baby last week, which was cool. She talks, but she also babbles and talks gibberish a lot. Yet, she's very excited and smiling. She'll respond to me usually. She's very happy that we're there. I mean, she's still there in her head."

Audra and I agreed that even excited gibberish is a tremendous gift with this disease. I reminded her she was lucky and that most people I spoke to weren't in the same boat.

There's one particular topic that always brings out the inner Shara.

"One of her things is water. Water is like a universal word. I don't know why we can't figure that out, but she says, 'I gotta go to the water.'"

The concept of water has become a constant theme throughout Shara's ordeal. For Audra, that theme also reminded her of the career she left behind. Audra's golf career centered around avoiding sand traps and water on the course.

She spent her entire life training her mind to see the water as a mile-wide roadblock from the pristine greens. In Florida, she made water her sanctuary and home, finally mastering treating one body of water as an enemy and the immense ocean as pleasure. Sadly, she sacrificed her career, life in the sun, and the safety net of a promising career for Shara's care. Audra told me that it was well worth it.

On a recent trip to Ocean City, Maryland, Audra watched Shara lying in 80-degree weather, bundled in towels because she's always chilly, smiling at the birds overhead. At that moment, near the water, Shara's anxiety and fear washed away. As Audra watched her mom find peace, she remembered something Shara told her as a child that put her desire for the water into perspective.

Thinking back to when she was ten or eleven, Audra said. "We were sitting on the beach in the dark, and she started crying. She was like, you know, 'I hope one day that the three of you find a passion as strong as my passion for this place on the beach.'"

"That's good that you remember after all those years," I said.

"On that recent trip, it all came back around for me. It's crazy that she still knows that's her happy place."

"It's remarkable that something like that sticks in your brain. At the time, you probably didn't even think it was important," I told her.

Timing means nothing without the reasons behind chasing the clock. Audra often finds herself focusing time on uncovering the "why?" of dementia. She explained how she managed to handle the agony of watching time slip away from Shara by the hour by flipping the idea of time on its side. If there's one thing I've learned from the Optimistics, it's that time will affect individuals with Alzheimer's differently. You don't have to expect others to understand your tricks to slow down dementia's clock.

"You know, any little thing, time as grief comes in, you know, any little thing," Audra said, laughing at herself. Like I'm looking at this clock—I have this clock that I found on somebody's stoop for free, so I grabbed it. It's broken, but it's always set to 3:00 AM."

Audra smiled. Once again, time cannot escape the world around her.

"What happened at 3:00 AM?"

"My mom loves Matchbox Twenty and Rob Thomas. *3AM* is one of her favorite songs. So, my siblings and I got tattoos, a version of the number 3 to symbolize the three of us and the fact that three o'clock was the last time my mom could read on an analog clock."

Last year, Shara turned sixty-one. Part of the celebration included a cameo Audra bought for Shara with Rob Thomas and other members of Matchbox Twenty, wishing Shara a happy birthday. Showing Shara the video was a moment when Audra saw the joy in her mom the way she did on past birthdays. This year, however, they celebrated Shara's birthday at the Stella Maris Nursing Home, where she now lives.

"I can't ask your mom this, but how do you stay optimistic for you?" Before she could answer, I reminded her to be open even if her viewpoint wasn't positive.

"I've had trouble being positive my whole life. I've always been very negative, like worry-wort. I think what has kept me optimistic about this situation is, number one, like I said earlier, seeing the beauty of the disease. I'm learning my mom in a new light. The biggest thing I've learned is the relationships and connections I've created throughout, like the whole world on social media. Having this group of people and being able to help people who were also in the situation I was in 2018-2019 when I felt like we had nowhere to turn."

"What do you think is the biggest lesson you've learned from this whole thing?"

"I would say, every moment—it's so cheesy—but it truly does count in life. Your life gets turned upside down at the snap of a finger, but the world will keep going. Whether you feel like you're stuck in this one moment, you have to move on, and you have to not take that moment for granted. Every single second that I'm with my mom, I refuse to take any of it for granted."

Audra stopped to rethink her words, fearing they may be too deep. "I don't know. It sounds pretty cliché."

"No, no, it's not cliché at all," I told her. "It's just something very hard for our generation. People don't digest and just relax about that notion."

"I think if I wanted my mom to be remembered for something, it was probably how I described her; sitting on the beach with her three kids, telling us how passionate she is about the beach and life—and I was so proud to have her as my mom." Audra shrugged and added, "I don't know if that came out right."

"It came out perfectly."

"She was just my best friend. So, yeah, I appreciate that."

Audra shook her head again and sneaked out a devilish grin. "See, you didn't make me cry," she said, referring to my earlier comment that most people came to tears during my interviews. "I'm shaking a little bit, but I'm not crying," she added.

"All right, fine," I replied with sarcasm, rolling my eyes. "I'll accept defeat on this one." Then added, "But for the record, that's not my goal. It just ends up happening."

My joke allowed Audra to relax again. Before our meeting ended, we made plans to one day get out on the golf course so she could show me some secrets. In exchange, I could boost her ego by showing her what an awful slice I have. Regardless, I know we'll have a good time, and I'll cherish every moment.

At the time of publication, Shara still lives in an assisted living facility with the around-the-clock care she needs. Scott still visits nearly daily, as does Audra. She values every second with her mom, despite her fractured speech and missing family memories. Three AM will be a time that will forever resonate with Audra and her siblings, reminding them that their bond is timeless. Even when the time comes for Shara's clock to tick slowly into the night, none of them will ever be alone in the dark.

CHAPTER THIRTEEN

Chris and Linda

LIFE IN A FISHBOWL

"We grabbed each other's hands, and Chris asked the doctor, 'How long do I have?'"

Chris was fifty-four when he was diagnosed with dementia. However, the signs were there years prior. Chris was charming and charismatic and could talk to anyone. He built a successful career in sales that allowed his wife, Linda, to stay at home for decades and raise their three kids. As dedicated Chris was to his job, it was the first aspect of his life to fracture. Neither Chris nor Linda was ready for something like dementia at his age.

"Not Chris, no way. Look at him! He's the life of the party. He's well dressed, good looking, and makes a great living. Not Chris."

Those sentiments are shared. No one looks like they have dementia, and people diagnosed are the last ones to admit it. But when polish is put on the exterior, it doesn't mean the interior isn't still rusted. Deep down, Chris knew this, which is the trail that paves the way for one's ADRD journey. Chris's coworkers picked up the signs he covered with a confident smile.

The "gut punch," as Linda described upon hearing the diagnosis, changed everything. Not only was their family's health in question, but finances were also an immediate concern.

"Chris got diagnosed on March first, and I went to work on March fourth, after being a stay-at-home mom for twenty-some years."

*   *   *   *   *

Chris and Linda are staples in the YES group meetings and he can't go unnoticed because he looks like someone famous. The second I saw him, I spent the next four meetings trying to figure out which Hollywood leading man he resembled. Even now, when his steps are smaller and his fitness days are behind him, he looks like "someone." Chris's salty hair compliments his frosty stubble that goes from a goatee to a light beard, depending on his mood. Linda perfectly complements his red carpet vibes with thick blonde hair, a dazzling smile, and bright eyes. Together, they are the admiration of their friends.

Hearing how they met sounds like a Barry Levinson or John Walters screenplay. It was a toasty summer day in Charm City at Preakness Weekend, 1993. Amid the crowd was a twenty-eight year old gym rat who looked like he walked off a movie set. That was Chris. Everyone knew him and wanted to be around him, including Linda. At twenty-seven, she perfectly complimented Chris's celebrity good looks.

"He's definitely easy on the eyes," Linda said, still picturing the day they met. "So, that helps. That was the first attraction."

Of course, there was more to Chris than a good smile that won Linda's heart. "Chris's love for his family," Linda said, "is his calling card to this day."

"Getting to know him, he was kind, thoughtful, and loving. He's all about family. He also comes from a very tight family, one of five boys. And his character and his faith—I mean, he has a very deep faith, and he lives by it. That's admirable and attractive. Seeing how he is with his family and his parents and how he adores them and looks up to his dad and his mom, he loves his mother."

From the moment they met, Linda knew how Chris would treat her. He promised her a home life and delivered. He also assured her their boys would be gentlemen, respecting their family and faith, which also came true. Chris also did everything he could to ensure that Linda would not have to worry about anything other than family obligations. That pledge, however, was something Chris could not control.

*   *   *   *   *

Privately, Linda knew there was more to Chris's constant migraines than stress. Sadly, his father had Alzheimer's Dementia but wasn't diagnosed until he was in his seventies. Considering their mutual love for their family, Chris's parents moved in with them. Caring for someone with his condition at home gave Linda a hands-on introduction to the world of dementia. As Chris began to show signs, Linda started checking off the boxes.

When the two of them left the doctor's office and the message sunk in, Chris made another promise to Linda. "We decided we're going to do what we always do and forge ahead." Chris told Linda, "I just want to try to live as normal a life as I can."

Normal would be impossible to pinpoint. Every day with dementia is a new bag of concerns filled with unlikely outcomes no one can prepare for. For Chris, trying to keep things patterned would involve taking away his purpose, which, as a husband, father, and provider, is what he values most. As a result, Chris's new normal was anything but commonplace. Being in sales, Chris was used to visiting customers and discussing ways he could help them. Now Chris was asking Linda, "What am I? I can't do anything. What do I do?"

Linda searched for an answer, which did not come right away. Watching Chris search for a new meaning guided her to a plan that Chris could accept.

"I told Chris, his contribution is exposing this disease and helping others," which Chris has championed in his way today. Despite having a reshaped mission, Chris's acceptance wasn't overnight.

Individuals with YOD feel disconnected from the older demographic of dementia. It can skew their acceptance of their condition and keep them further isolated. Like others, Chris didn't feel comfortable in a room of people in their seventies and eighties, most in wheelchairs or accompanied by nurses, to speak openly about his battle. That was until he met Jim and the other Optimistics. Linda is friends with Jim's sister-in-law and connected with Jim's wife, Terri. Chris joined the group, welcomed with open arms.

Discovering the Optimistics through mutual contacts was more than just a coincidence in Linda's eyes. "I think this was placed here for us. God places that here. Here's your help."

Finally, Chris had people he could relate to, and Linda had spouses she could confide in as well. That, as she told me, was the real missing piece. Dementia is a disease that people whisper about and handle with uncertainty, which often results in personal relationships falling by the wayside. As much as the Optimistics provided a place to come together, Linda began to feel that her world was like a fishbowl. In the fishbowl is the community that the support group provides, but people swam past her and Chris outside that fishbowl.

While others are going on lavish vacations, Chris and Linda live in a world blocked into days that are only around the corner. While their peers review retirement plans for ten or fifteen years down the road, Chris was forced into retirement a decade and a half too early. While others discuss their children getting married and spending their final years with grandchildren running around the house, Chris and Linda's views as grandparents are drastically different. Their boys also know this but must swim at their own pace. Regardless of the speed at which Linda and Chris step towards "normalcy," they remind each other of their vows, with promises of being there for each other still being kept.

Finding their own normal still left Chris questioning how people would look back at him when he was no longer here to hug or kiss his loved ones. Linda and Chris had that conversation many times, and she went back to his image of always being a provider. She connected his love for family with his passion for music when Chris pinpointed precisely how he would like to be remembered.

"Chris loves the band, RUSH. We even made shirts for the Alzheimer's Walk that said 'RUSH For The Cure'. It's our team name with the Alzheimer's Association. He told me what he wanted for his final days and thought of a song by RUSH called, *The Garden*. It sums him up perfectly in how he wants to be remembered: respected and loved."

After we spoke, I listened to *The Garden* on repeat for two hours and thought of Chris. Even while I write this chapter, it's playing. The last line reminded me of a story Linda told about Chris that was wildly unexpected while they were going on one of their long walks.

"We don't have a lot of big conversations because it's difficult for him to get thoughts and words out. But we were walking one day, and he asked me, 'Where do you live?' which surprised me."

Although the reality of their conversation highlighted Chris's confusion, it sent them back in time to when they first met. She held his hand, then rubbed his arm. "I was like, oh my, here we go. I started thinking I could either sit here and cry or go with it. I decided to go with it."

Linda recalled the conversation as if it just happened.

I said, "I live in the neighborhood, back up the street here," pointing toward their home.

Keeping the conversation going, Linda asked Chris the same question. "I grew up in Catonsville," he said, which was correct.

Chris then asked Linda, "Where did you grow up?"

Linda responded.

Then, the family man Linda loved so much shined through. He asked her, "Are your parents still alive?"

"No. Unfortunately, my mom passed away last year, and my dad passed away a year before that," she replied.

"Oh. I'm sorry," Chris said.

They continued their walk, holding hands the entire time. Linda said she asked him about his parents. "No. My dad passed, but my mom's around," he told her.

Then, Chris stopped and looked into Linda's eyes, "You would love my mom," he told her. Then, he added, "You know what? I think she'd like you too."

Linda hoped the moment would never end.

She laid her head against Chris's shoulder as they walked side by side, holding hands, just as they did in their twenties, then later when pushing their boys in strollers. Being people of faith, Chris and Linda view life as a blessing, regardless of how small their fishbowl becomes daily. Still, though, there is optimism for Linda.

"Optimism means doing your best, and you see just that. You see good in other people too," she began, "you look on then try to look on the brighter side of every day because if you don't have the light, you're in the dark, and you do your best."

If you're wondering, Chris's mom does like Linda. How could she not? For Chris and Linda, hope remains. It has become the soil that nurtures their garden, which, despite Chris's dementia, continues to thrive with love, laughter, and a charming grin from one heck of a handsome man.

CHAPTER FOURTEEN

Glenn and Val

THE SINGER AND THE SONG

"Hope and fear walk side by side." That is how Val talks about the future of her husband, Glenn.

Today, Glenn and Val walk arm in arm into the darkness, forbidding the light to dim on the man Glenn used to be. Rather than let shadows block their visions of a comfortable future together, Val's smile lights up with confidence about Glenn beating the clock of Father Time.

When you first meet Val, you can't help but like her. There's an unexplainable pull she has. There's also a glow about her that creates a sense of warmth when she speaks. Dignified and relaxed, it's another reason Glenn fell in love with Val from the moment he saw her at a happy hour event. Although they have a twelve-year age difference and were initially just friends, Glenn wasted no time connecting with Val once she invited him out to hear her band at a local nightclub.

She was a singer in a band at a local nightclub who captivated the room with her voice. Glenn was one of those people watching in the crowd as she closed her eyes to hit notes he had never heard before. Val remembers when she first saw Glenn at happy hour weeks before. He was with his brothers and it was clear there was an interest between them. However, that was all there was at the time.

Glenn's a hard guy to miss too. He's six-foot-three, fit and trim like a track star with an air of confidence that always brings out the introvert in others. Val said, "He was always the life of the party. He was very engaging, a great conversationalist, and people loved being around him."

Val described Glenn as a natural leader, which showed in his work. For decades, he worked in the federal government. Along with climbing the ladder of success, his personality earned him the Regional President for the Blacks In Government, a national non-profit organization dating back to 1975. He would even take his daughters to meetings when they were younger to learn more about the fantastic work his team members had accomplished.

Glenn traveled nationwide to attend conferences and speak at seminars. He remained a constant advocate for careers in the public sector. His fondness for travel even allowed Glenn to dabble in the world of being a part-time travel agent. When people needed an idea for a dream vacation, Glenn was the one they went to for guidance. In every aspect of Glenn's world, people felt safe and secure in his presence, which Val found to be an attractive quality in a partner.

Val admits her nervousness in jumping from a family friend to a romantic partner. She knew that once they crossed that line, it would be for good, and nearly twenty years later, they know the timing was right. Over the past few years, Glenn has become intimately familiar with time. Not only is time important due to his dementia, but Glenn suffered tremendous loss before his diagnosis. He has three girls from previous relationships. His oldest, Valaicia, and then twins, Sharice and Letrice. Sadly, tragedy sent Glenn's world into a spiral when Letrice was killed as a result of a car accident when she was only twenty-two. Glenn was hit with a level of grief that he never knew was imaginable. To this day, Val said Glenn doesn't like to talk about the accident. The incident brought Glenn and his other daughters closer together. As a result, they became amazing big sisters to Jaelyn, the daughter Glenn and Val had in 2008.

The irony of trying to capture moments can play tricks on your mind regarding the "what ifs?" life throws your way. For instance, have you ever met someone and wondered, "What if I met them years ago? How would that have changed my life?" Be it professional or personal, certain people become friends relatively quickly, and you feel like you've known them forever. This was my situation with Glenn. Over a decade ago our paths crossed, but we never connected.

The day I met Glenn and Val at a support group meeting was not the first time I had seen him. Glenn and I used to work together at the same government agency. Although our work areas never intersected I knew of him because he stood out.

I remember a tall, clean-cut man, always in a fine suit, sporting an ear-to-ear smile, swaying through the sea of employees with handshakes and hugs. I'd see him in the cafeteria, the hallway, or an all-hands conference. We never spoke one-on-one, but I remembered Glenn for some cosmic reason that can only be a sign of the presence he carries. When he walked into the meeting with Val, I couldn't help but introduce myself right away.

Glenn didn't remember me, but he made me feel like we'd known each other forever. Val was just as surprised about the coincidence, and later on, she would tell me how she was so proud of his career. I told her he made it look like he respected his role. I didn't know what he did but if I were looking in a crowd for someone to turn to for answers, it would have been that sharp-dressed man in the hallway.

Looking back at how many times our paths ran parallel as strangers, I realize now that I witnessed some of the most challenging times of Glenn's life. It was also the same year he found Val to refill his heart with life's passion after tremendous loss. I reminded Val of this when we first sat down to speak about Glenn. She believes there is a more spiritual angle to our meeting at this point in Glenn's life and the devotion I have to share his and other Optimistics' stories with the world. Although I don't consider myself overly religious, when talking to Val I become a believer. Val learned to listen to her inner voice.

Being twelve years younger than Glenn, Val was aware that statistically he could have health issues before her, but no one ever thought it would be this soon. In hindsight, Val said, the signs were there for many years before the official diagnosis.

"When I think back to little things I saw, I could have known then, but Alzheimer's was not even in consideration."

Many YOD individuals try to hide signs of their dementia, which buys them more time to shelter their pain from the public. Along with his youthfulness, Glenn always presented well, which is another way YOD individuals mask their illness, even to themselves.

She said, "He always dressed well and paid a lot of attention to how he looked, especially at work."

I agreed with her, having seen it firsthand for years. I told Val that when I met them for the first time, Glenn seemed to have everything under control, almost to the point that he didn't belong in the group meetings. He is still in impeccable shape and despite a sweet tooth, Glenn remains remarkably fit, with what looks like softballs for biceps. I was wrong, but I could still see how Glenn's calm personality could have bought him more time than most. Whether it was work or around friends, Glenn was always making jokes, smiling wide, and ready for a hug, with his long arms wrapping everyone up like a cozy blanket. Although his charisma may have overshadowed the signs of dementia to his coworkers or friends, nothing was getting past Val. As with every case between a spouse and an Optimistic, the partner always knows first.

"Was there one event that made you question things?"

"Yes," Val said. "One day he was supposed to have an appointment and he didn't leave."

"Did he call you or tell you he wasn't going?"

"No, I saw it for myself on our security cameras. He forgot he was supposed to go."

Glenn was caught, and this was the real moment when Val realized there was more to his forgetfulness than he had led on. After some arm twisting, Glenn finally agreed to see a doctor. Finally, Val would have answers to Glenn's condition, and they could tackle it together. To Val's surprise, the appointment did not go as anticipated.

"We went to the doctor and the doctor said he was fine," Val said, still frustrated at that day. His doctor did mention that maybe he should get an assessment for his memory. Glenn kind of threw his hands up and said, 'See,' he said 'I'm fine. I'm fine so no need for an assessment.'"

The doctor's passive reply that Glenn was fine didn't convince Val. She wanted the doctor to definitively tell him that he needed to see a neurologist for an assessment. After all, the doctor gave him the green light. In his mind, the issue was over, but to Val, this was just the start of something bigger. Since Glenn held onto the doctor's comments that he was fine, it was nearly a year before Val finally got Glenn assessed by a neurologist because he refused to go. This time, things were different.

"It was hard to hear the neurologist talk about dementia," Val said. "It didn't feel real."

"How did Glenn act?"

"In that moment he was shocked. He exhaled deeply then sat back in his chair." Driving home Glenn said, "It is what it is."

Val told me about the first days after the diagnosis. The variety of emotions that went through her mind were all over the spectrum. First, how Glenn must have felt in that moment of hearing the diagnosis. Second, she thought about Glenn's older children and their daughter together, Jaelyn, who was around twelve at the time of his diagnosis.

—*How do you tell your teenage daughter their father has dementia?*

—How do you handle your child asking about the future?

"How *do* you talk about the future?" I asked.
"Glenn doesn't like to talk about the future."

*   *   *   *   *

Jaelyn The Brave

The expression "They don't make them like that any-more" should be dedicated to Jaelyn. When I spoke to her, I quickly realized she was unique. She is not only one of the most mature teenagers I've ever met, but she has the soul of a saint and the compassion of Mother Teresa. Jaelyn also has Glenn's bright smile that runs the width of her entire face when she talks about her father. Val calls Jaelyn and Glenn "two peas in a pod" and says everything is a "yes" to Jaelyn. Being Daddy's Girl isn't something Jaelyn takes for granted. At only fifteen she's poised, composed, and knows exactly what's happening with her father. Not only is she aware of dementia, she's become a champion, educating other young people about the disease.

I told Jaelyn that my daughter, Maddy, is the same age, and she lit up at the coincidence. I see the similarities be-tween them which makes me more emotional when she speaks. Every time Jaelyn says, "My dad," it hits me differ-ently than other children of Optimistics. Putting myself in Glenn's shoes, the possibility that my daughter would have to go through what Jaelyn so elegantly has had to is a jarring notion to try and absorb. Being so young, it's hard for other people her age who aren't in her shoes to understand what it's like to watch a parent go through Alzheimer's. Although she doesn't shy away from talking about Glenn's condition if asked, she learned early on that his situation is not something many young people can relate to in their own lives.

"My dad has always been a very funny person," Jaelyn said delicately. "He always knows how to trip people up and make them laugh. There's a lot of times where, if I wasn't feeling the best, he'd always end up telling me some story or a joke that would just make me feel better."

She smiled at the memory.

Her smile is infectious in the same way Val's gentle, singsong tone is and just as inviting as when Glenn wraps his long arms around you for a hug.

"He's always been the life of the party, someone that's a very optimistic person, very lighthearted, and very fun."

"How have things changed from his personality aspect or interaction with him since the diagnosis?"

"His personality hasn't changed much, but he has become very persistent. He was always a stubborn person. If he had an idea, he'd stick with that idea. With the diagnosis, now he's stubborn about things that he shouldn't be doing."

"In what ways?"

"Well, he likes to go on walks. And if we tell him it's not good weather or it's too far, then he still goes anyway because that's what he wants to do and he's going to do it."

"How old were you when you first heard about his diagnosis?"

"He was diagnosed in 2020, and I was in seventh grade, so I was about eleven."

"Did you understand what that meant?"

"I had heard about it before but had to look at it more. I had the basics, and since then, I've been researching more specific things related to my dad."

As her research explained, Jaelyn learned it's best to keep Glenn's mind active. Together, they'll work on puzzles and play chess. He has taken to both activities with positive energy, allowing her to sneak in even more father-daughter moments she can hold onto. Recently, Val bought a book on chess so all three of them could learn together. Whether it's through mental stimulation or laughter from a good movie, dementia has shown her she must embrace those good moments. Unable to predict when his condition will devolve, Jaelyn is dedicated to being present.

"Do you think about the later years or about the college years coming up?"

"I have thought about it somewhat. I'm definitely going to college. I want to do something in the medical field too. I'm also thinking about double majoring in nursing and neuroscience. I am interested in the brain and in Young-Onset Dementia."

I'm often at a loss when talking to Jaelyn. At no point during our conversation did she lose her composure or falter when talking about Glenn. I can see a lot of Val in her responses, and when she discusses the uncertain road ahead, she does so with confidence. In my Optimistics journey of interviewing family, I'm always surprised by how they answer the topic of remaining optimistic.

"Well, since the book is called *The Optimistics* and about how you look at optimism in the face of this disease, can you find a level of optimism?"

With Jaelyn being so involved in the YOD community and a spokesperson, her response was beyond what I expected.

She tilted her head in thought and smiled once again. "My mom taught me that the person that they used to be doesn't really exist anymore and they're fading away. So, instead of holding on to who they used to be, and then wondering why they're not like that anymore, you have to let go of that. You have to move on because it's okay, this is who they are now."

I shook my head and said, "You're fifteen, but you sound like you're thirty-five." I remain in awe of her take on Glenn to this day.

She thanked me; however, I owe her all the gratitude I can hold.

"Things are going to be difficult," she added, "but there's always things that you can learn in the process. Like things I'm learning about my dad—new things I wouldn't have learned. But I have to let go of that and accept that this is who he is now. Regardless of who he is and how he acts, he's still my father, and I'm still going to love him. Holding on to that, even though he's not the same, he's still my father."

As if Jaelyn already spun around my mind, she layered even more intensity to her already deep insight, "I think that the whole idea of optimism is just to know that there is better and that it will get better."

With a stable and steady daughter like Jaelyn in the house, someone may say that Val and Glenn have it better than most. In the way of emotional maturity and a realistic approach to Alzheimer's, yes, Val and Glenn are fortunate. Yet no level of stability can keep you guarded from the onslaught of Alzheimer's sporadic blows. Glenn's stubbornness is one of the areas where his reality gets blurred due to his condition. As Jaelyn mentioned, Glenn loves to walk outside but needs help determining the manageable lengths or conditions.

"I find that there is this independence factor that comes with many who have YOD," I said to Val, to which she nodded in agreement. "It's built into our DNA that men are supposed to provide for the family and then suddenly that's gone. It hits our egos. I wonder if that's a part he misses now?"

Val knows precisely what I mean, and she's seen it almost daily firsthand. Glenn is obsessed with walking to the bank or the convenience store. Even if he goes to the bank to take out twenty dollars, doing so is ingrained into his self-image. There are times when a bank manager will call Val and tell her Glenn is trying to make a withdrawal. Val is torn between allowing Glenn a level of independence that satisfies his ego and keeping him safe. She also mentioned that he's crossing traffic at all hours on these walks.

Although Glenn hasn't had a problem yet, there is a general fear of him losing his cognition while walking across traffic. Still, how do you tell your grown-up husband that he can't do something simple like going for a walk? Val battles with the length of Glenn's independence, and there are times when Glenn's persistence pushes Val to the edge of concern.

One situation that concerned her the most was when she found Glenn in their bedroom packing his clothes. Val heard shuffling coming from upstairs, which sounded unusual. When she entered their bedroom she saw Glenn took all of his clothes out of his drawers and their closet, then tossed them into a duffel bag. She immediately asked him what was going on.

"I'm going home," he said as he piled random clothes into his bag.

"Where was he going?"

Val told me there is a family house from his mother where Glenn used to live when he was younger. People from all stretches of his family would constantly be over the house, which came to be referred to as the "family house." Glenn and the girls have been back to visit many times. For an unknown reason that day, he determined that his house with Val was not his real home. Val held his hands and calmly explained he was already home. Glenn, however, was still adamant about leaving. To her amazing credit, she eventually talked him back to the present and then distracted him from the idea of leaving. She still fears the topic may come up again and how she'll have to overcome that obstacle.

Patterns like this are common in individuals with dementia. In a previous story, one YOD individual thought they were trapped in a prison when in reality they lived in a very comfortable house with their daughter. Other people I spoke to said their loved one recalled a specific moment in their life from the past as happening in the present, which can confuse a person with dementia as separating fiction from reality. In all situations, I can't imagine the anxiety the YOD individual is going through when they feel threatened by their surroundings.

When Val retold the story of that day, I felt for her, Jaelyn, and Glenn. I tried to put myself in Glenn's mind, feeling that he didn't belong in his house or wasn't supposed to be there. The panic that took over his body enough to gather all of his belongings must have been frightening. His mind told him to flee, escape, and return to a home he once knew, even if that meant leaving Val. Thankfully, she dared to bring him back down and remind him of the house they built together as a family.

Glenn spoke to me about the idea of togetherness and family at lunch one day. I asked him what being a part of the Optimistics community has meant to him. His speech was slower and he struggled to use the right words. Like a person with a severe stutter, he knows what he wants to say, but getting the thought out of his mouth takes great effort.

He tapped his fingers together in a tented position. His lips tightened as he worked to form his words and I waited patiently while he did. Then he said, "Togetherness."

"Togetherness?"

Glenn smiled. "I feel a sense of togetherness. All of us care so much about each other," he said. "We're all in this together."

I felt a weight of relief left his voice when he finished speaking. A moment like that makes remaining optimistic for your loved ones so important. At any time their mind can make enough room for their heart to take over and return them to who they once were. Glenn used togetherness to describe the Optimistics, and I humbly use that word when referring to Glenn, Val, Jaelyn, and all of their children.

Togetherness isn't just a concept. It's a practice, and as a family, they can love Glenn for who he was and honor the man he is today. It's not easy, but it's also not unrealistic when you have Glenn's strong family support in and outside of the home, combined with the strength of the Optimistics.

As Jaelyn said in our interview, "As long as you can take a couple of deep breaths and think and react appropriately, then it's all going to be okay."

CHAPTER FIFTEEN

Lorinn

A BICYCLE IN THE SHOWER

"After I was diagnosed, my mother asked me, 'What does this mean?' I told her, 'This means I'll probably die before you do.'"

When I was in college studying art, I had a professor who was every bit the artist I imagined a professional painter to be, as if I drew her myself. She was from France and spoke several different languages. She donned worn-in jeans with paint stains and a t-shirt as if she didn't have time to look like a college professor. She liked the same music as we did, laughed with all the students, told wild stories of her travels, and supported our work. She had something positive to offer during critiques, which is usually the tough honesty portion of an art class. Even if you could tell she didn't truly understand the intent behind the work, she found a way to give positive feedback and guidance on technique.

One woman in our class was in her fifties and took that class for personal enjoyment. She generally got along with everyone but usually kept to herself. Having the freedom of fun rather than a graded structure, regardless of the assignment, she would always paint in abstract. We painted a fruit bowl to exact detail, and she did it with large, elaborate circles of various colors puddled together. When we had to paint a nude body, the other students and I focused on movement and shadows, while her paintings looked like Picasso's initial sketches, but with circles. However, after many weeks of watching this woman float past every project with an abstract escape of whatever her mind told her, one student spoke out during a critique session.

With teenage frustration in his tone, he challenged, "What is it?"

Sure, we all thought the same thing, but I immediately felt terrible for the woman. That's not how we were taught to critique, and "What is it?" does not benefit anyone's development, as is the intention of a critique. Then, the relatively swift and cool teacher spun his comment on a dime and said, "It's paint on canvas."

The guy quickly shut up.

Those four words changed my mind when explaining my work to people outside the art world who never understood me. Her phrase was a slap in the face of anyone who doesn't try to embrace what an outsider sees as someone's heart and only looks at the surface of anything or anyone. When I met Lorinn for the first time, I told her this story, hoping my anecdote about her condition could be something she could use as well. After all, if there is any person I've met through this book who sees things differently than anyone else, it's her.

At fifty-two, Lorinn was diagnosed with dementia just two years before the time I first met her. Only four-foot-ten inches, she hardly goes unnoticed, having earned and enjoyed a reputation for being feisty, comical, flirtatious, and not afraid to make an inappropriate joke. She reminds me of Elaine from *Seinfeld*, who, combined with that one friend we all have, is always the best guest at a wedding. One minute, she's entertaining us about a doctor's appointment gone awry, then commenting, "That's what she said," during a conversation at a group therapy session. Even with her diagnosis, she hasn't lost a step in her personality, especially considering her condition of dementia is one of the rarest in the world.

Lorin has Posterior Cortical Atrophy (PCA), and with her condition, language is usually the first to go, followed by the behavioral variant Frontotemporal Dementia (FTD). According to Dr. Karen Dionesotes, MD, MPH, a YES group volunteer who received her degree in Geriatric Psychiatry at Johns Hopkins University, FTD causes behavioral changes and is the primary presenting symptom, causing language deficits. Out of all cases that fall under the umbrella of ADRD, there are only 50,000 to 60,000 people with the behavioral variant FDA and PCA in the entire United States. Due to its rarity, finding the proper resources for PCA is challenging, and meeting others like them in their community is not common. When you factor in the consistency of depression and loneliness felt by individuals with dementia, people like Lorinn are even more isolated because of her unique condition.

As an active support group volunteer, Dr. Dionesotes has known Lorinn since she joined the group. She is keen on discovering ways to help PCA individuals manage their illness but admits there is still a lot to uncover, which is unfortunate for anyone with this condition.

"There are multiple types of PCA. There are those that have an inability to express themselves and those who cannot understand language," Dr. Dionesotes began. "They present very differently because those who cannot express themselves have a lot of word-finding difficulties and they get frustrated with their inability to grasp words. Those who cannot understand language may nod along to whatever you're saying and are saying complete sentences, but none of it makes sense."

Adding more complexity to Lorinn's situation is that her specific form of PCA not only contorts her depth perception but also creates life-like images that aren't there at all. At the first support group meeting where Lorinn was in attendance, she told a story about how she went on a walk in a nearby park and became convinced that two people were fooling around in the open.

"I could see it right in front of me. Right there! Two people, clearly making out," she said with a cheeky smile. "Then I got closer, and it was just two bushes."

She was adamant, though, that what she saw was reality. During our first video call together, she stopped twice in the middle of a conversation.

At minute thirty-three, she cut me off, asking, "Are you on a bicycle?"

"Me? No. I'm right here. At a table."

"Oh, it looked like you were on a bicycle," she said, laughing at herself.

Around the fifty-five-minute mark, she asked me, "Wait, are you in the shower?"

By this time, we had been joking enough that I understood how PCA could alter her vision and said, "Actually, yes, I am. I'm on a bicycle, in the shower. I'm very talented."

We both laughed at one another.

"It's this damn PCA, man, I'm telling you," she said.

The situation was hilarious, but the difficulties of her brain convincing her eyes that something was in front of her could also be life-threatening.

"I had no idea what was wrong with me at first. When I was driving, I would end up breaking right before the car in front of me, and I almost hit them when I should have just slowed down like you're supposed to. But in many cases, I stopped right behind the person in front of me, like a foot away, and I knew I had to figure this out."

Like others with dementia, driving is usually the first luxury to be stripped away; however, Lorinn wasn't as concerned with driving as she was with getting dressed every day. One sign of PCA is when people can't put their clothes on properly, even though they know exactly how it's supposed to be worn. With the delivery of a stand-up comedian, she explained her troubles with getting dressed. I had no problem with her tone.

"Can I curse?" she asked.

"Of course! Curse away."

Lorinn felt relieved. "One day, I had this blouse that had spaghetti strings in the back, so it was open in the back. I know which side of the shirt is the front and the back, but I can't figure out how to do it," she began. I could see the frustration in her facial expressions, recalling that day. "I knew that was the back of the shirt, but I couldn't get the fucking thing on!"

She laughed, which made me laugh.

"I laid it on my bed and said, 'You got this; you can do this!' But it didn't work. Then, I got even more pissed and shouted, 'I'm going to put you on, you mother fucker!'"

In another situation, Lorinn was at a restaurant with her father. Toward the end of the evening, when she tried putting on her jacket, her PCA did not allow her arms to reach the sleeves. Frustrated, she stared at the jacket and flung it about her body, but it wasn't working. Seeing that she was growing impatient, her father intervened.

"I'm trying to put my jacket on, and then my dad goes, 'Lorinn, you have to put your arms in the sleeves,' and I lost it! I shouted at him, 'I fucking know where the fucking sleeves are, Dad!'"

Beneath the humor, I could sense the defeat she still feels when someone tries to help her. She knew her father meant well, but for her, it was a reminder that not only did no one else understand what she was going through, but she didn't either. It was during a doctor's appointment with her gynecologist that Lorinn found the answers she needed.

"I thought all of this was maybe from menopause or something. I'm explaining what was happening, and then my doctor asks, 'Do you have problems putting your clothes on?' and I said, 'Yes! Yes, I do!' It was the first time anyone had asked me that," she said, wide-eyed in excitement. "Then he said to me, 'You have to go see a neurologist right away,' and so I did."

Other symptoms began to develop that were more painful than getting dressed. When looking at a photograph of her nineteen-year-old son, she said she couldn't recognize him. As a mother, it broke her heart. Between driving, issues with clothes, and remembering the faces of people close to her, Lorinn's upbeat personality would soon be challenged. When Lorinn received her diagnosis of Alzheimer's Dementia (AD) and PCA, her world shattered.

"I was furious," she recalled. "I yelled at the doctors, at their staff, anyone. I didn't want to believe it. I was so young—too young."

Lorinn's blunt frustration and honesty towards her diagnosis were similarly expressed when she had to tell her parents.

"I imagine the conversation with your parents was rough?"

She smiled, now able to laugh at how comfortable she was telling people about her condition. "After I was diagnosed, my mother asked me, 'What does this mean?' and I told her, 'This means I'll probably die before you do.'"

There's not much more to say after that, and Lorinn did it purposely. Like ripping a bandage off; quick, easy, and direct is the only way to present her wounds to the public. She knows there is no hiding her condition, and as I said already, she can't resist a good punchline.

"Wow, you didn't hold back, did you?"

"What's the point? We're all adults, and she knows something wasn't right. Now I have a title for it."

Thinking outside her parents, she also had to tell her two sons, Devin, twenty-six and Mason, twenty-four. Both discussions were grueling. Although it would be hard for her parents to hear, they have been around dementia before. However, for her sons, their mom's entire journey would be something any child finds difficult comprehend at first. For the first time during our meeting, Lorinn hesitated to have a good sense of humor about her condition when discussing Devin and Mason.

"Do they understand?"

"They get it, but..." she trailed off.

She's proud of how her boys have helped her throughout her condition. Devin, who lives in New Jersey, calls all the time, and visits as much as he can. Lorinn told me that he came in to help her with her taxes, since PCA has affected her ability to read. Mason is her right hand man, keeping the house together, and doing her laundry. He's also her go-to driver, whenever she needs a ride. He does it happily, no matter how far or how long her appointment may take. When Mike isn't available, Mason takes her to the monthly including the support group meetings, despite living forty-five minutes away.

One meeting, when I arrived late, I saw him in the parking lot, watching his phone in his car. I wanted to introduce myself, hoping my voice could connect with him on another level. Then, I thought about Lorinn. Having met many children—from teenagers to retirees—of individual's with dementia, there is no set timetable for a child to embrace their parent's condition. I remember walking by his car and waving rather than knocking on the window for a conversation.

Despite her sense of humor towards life, it took a while for her to grasp her future living with PCA and YOD. She read enough material and met with dozens of specialists to

206 | RICHIE FRIEMAN

realize there was no escaping her condition. Even worse, her "double dose of dementia," as she calls it, means her chances of longevity are even shorter. However, her original upbeat character slowly found its way back to the surface. Although still fearful of her future, she welcomed each day as she did before her diagnosis. Lorinn even went back to dating after being divorced for several years.

I thought twice about asking her for more details about her dating life as someone with dementia, but it was a door she opened, and I had to visit. "Can I ask you something I hope doesn't come out wrong?"

"Sure."

"How long do you wait to tell people about your unique situation?"

Lorinn waved her hand. "Please. I tell them right away. Why hide it? They're going to find out."

"Yeah, especially if you come to dinner with your shirt on backwards," I said.

"You're right!" she laughed. "But no, I say it upfront. I went on Bumble and met a great guy named Mike. He accepts me and loves me for who I am, for as long as that is."

I met Mike at one of the YES meetings, and if there is such a thing as a perfect match, it's Lorinn and Mike. He is a barrel-chested rock of a man who looks like a mix between a nose tackle and a bouncer at a rowdy college bar with the disposition of a teddy bear. His broad smile fills whatever room he's in, especially when talking about Lorinn.

Lorinn said she told Mike that she doesn't know how her illness will advance and to what degree, and Mike has been all in from the beginning. One night, though, Mike went with her to a support group session (not with YES), and after listening to everyone's story, he told her, "I didn't like what I heard."

To this day, Mike is by Lorinn's side, holding her hand through the ups and downs of her illness.

Between her unique sense of humor and the love she's surrounded by, I assumed her approach towards optimism had a similar boost of "Lorinn-positivity." Ironically, her take on optimism is more based on a spiritual acknowledgment.

"I think about this a lot," she said.

"Optimism?"

"Yes, and about this whole thing. I tell myself it's nothing I did to deserve this, it's not my fault, and I don't have any control over it. So, I'm not going just to lay around and cry about it," she said. Then, added, "I've done that already."

Her statement led us to speak about the darkness that others have felt while going through dementia. She admitted she had spent a long time in fear and had yet to find a way out of that hole. "I have a life to live, and I'm going to live it. I'm not going to dwell on the timetable."

I told her I love her attitude, not only now but how she carries her optimism to the meetings and to the AD community at large. Lorinn nodded along and smiled. Then, she leaned into the camera and threw her hands out.

"I don't want to spend my life laying in bed wondering what people are going to say at my funeral."

Every time someone I speak to discusses their funeral, I get uncomfortably emotional. No matter how positive they are about death, thinking of their absolute final day is a topic I still have trouble discussing. Through this process, I had let down walls of my own regarding vulnerabilities; however, everyone I spoke to felt at ease, and we became like family rather quickly. When I think about their futures, reminding myself about having to attend their funerals one day is something I'm not ready to accept. I can't imagine a world where Lorinn isn't hopping around the room with a sarcastic comment or asking for a refill of wine.

I continue to see Lorinn at the monthly support group meetings, and she welcomes me with a big hug as she folds into my chest like a toddler. "You good?" she asks. "Everything good with you?" she says happily. As I am used to seeing her and other Optimistics at the meetings, I take mental notes about how they have changed month to month. Some people walk slower, others are more timid or reserved, and sadly, most need reminders about who they are talking to.

Several months after our initial interview, I saw her at a support group meeting as usual. As always, we said hello, she gave me a big hug, we chatted for a bit, and then went on to catch up with other people before the group session began. No more than five minutes after I spoke to Lorinn, she sat down next to me at a table.

When I saw her walking my way, I pulled out a chair for her and said, "Here, join me," I said, patting the open seat.

Lorinn sat down and then tilted her head. "Who are you again?"

At first, I thought she was kidding, especially since I had just spoken to her. I quickly realized she wasn't, and this was the first time she had forgotten me. More importantly, it was also within minutes of talking to one another.

"I'm Richie."

She nodded and pointed her finger. "Wait, I do know you."
I smiled. "You do. We're friends."

Lorinn pointed her finger at me as if I jogged her memory for the moment. "Ah, you're right! Richie," she said. "Yup, I figured we were friends."

As I finished this chapter, Lorinn and Mike were still together. She still lights up the room of every support group meeting and whips out hilarious one-liners whenever possible. Lorinn is still fighting day in and day out to rally her body against the side effects of PCA...and celebrates every time a shirt goes on the right way.

CHAPTER SIXTEEN

Andy and Laurie

BASEBALL, BRUCE, AND TRAVELING

" **A**ndy said many times, 'I'm going to be the first person who survives this. I'm going to be that person,' and I wanted to support that for him."

Laurie and Andy hit it off on their first date, a blind date facilitated by their dogs. Laurie said that even though their dogs didn't get along at first, their "doggy date" was just what she needed. As a single mother, Laurie saw a caring father for her daughter, Amanda, and a lifelong partner in Andy. He was gentle, wise, compassionate, and so easy to be with. Andy found in Laurie a partner he could be himself with, who shared the same values and who made him smile and laugh—a lot. That date was nearly twenty-five years ago.

"We had very similar values in things that were important in the world. The kindness, compassion, and love were the same, so it was a good fit. Andy was just so loving, warm, and embracing of Amanda that it quickly became sort of a threesome," she said, reflecting on the fond memory of her daughter embracing Andy as a father figure early on.

Andy and Amanda embraced their lives together. Very early on, they would go on Saturday adventures, just the two of them, to the park, minor league baseball games, or the library. Amanda loved traveling on Andy's shoulders and wearing his old baseball jerseys. A favorite memory of Andy's was the time he babysat for Amanda and agreed to have his nails painted green. He wore the nail polish proudly to work for a week. It didn't matter to him how the other partners in his CPA firm and clients reacted to his nails. He only cared that it made Amanda happy.

Laurie still laughs at the day they told Amanda that Andy was moving in with them. "When we sat down to tell Amanda or really to ask Amanda how she would feel if Andy moved in, she immediately ran and opened up closet space. Then she started running around the house, telling him all the places that he could put his stuff."

Two years later, in 2001, Andy and Laurie married. She was thirty-eight, and he was forty, with this being the first marriage for each of them. Continuing Andy's deep connection with Amanda, he proudly wore the badge of stepfather. However, before their wedding, Laurie and Andy wanted to ensure Amanda was comfortable with the "title" Andy would hold in the family. Being conscious that Amanda never had a father figure in her life, Laurie and Andy give Amanda a list of options, but Amanda already has her mind made up.

"I like Daddy," Amanda said with a bubbly smile.

Their family of three quickly developed into four when their daughter Jaden was born, not including the three dogs they shared. Life for Laurie, Andy, Amanda, and Jaden was beautiful for quite a while. Unfortunately, challenges in the marriage surfaced over time. They agreed to separate in 2012 with the hope that some time apart would allow for a rebuilding of the relationship. They went to counseling, communicated every day, and worked to stay connected as a foursome through family dinners and activities. Laurie and Andy continued to share family responsibilities and the girls' well-being remained a priority for them. Andy found an apartment close to their home so that he and the girls could see each other as often as they liked.

"The plan was to create a little bit of space with the idea that we will work on this. We're going to work on this. We're going to go to therapy," Laurie said. "We both felt very committed to working this through."

Andy's new address allowed him and Laurie to keep their distance but kept him close enough to see the kids whenever he wanted. On the day Andy was set to move into his new place, he planned to do so while Laurie was at work and the kids were in school. However, when Laurie came home that afternoon, Andy hadn't moved anything and was sitting in the family room watching TV like any other day of the week.

Laurie asked him what had happened, why he wasn't at his new apartment. He looked at her with a blank stare and said, "I forgot".

To this, Laurie responded, "Are you kidding? Why would you make one of the worst days of our lives more difficult?" Again, a blank stare.

"Did you think he was being stubborn?" I asked.

Laurie shook her head at the frustration she felt that day. "I just could not wrap my head around it."

In hindsight, Laurie identified many signs of Young-Onset Dementia. What seemed like a misstep in judgment or poor time management became "ah-ha" moments correlating to Andy's developing dementia. On Father's Day, a year before their separation, the family had plans to meet his parents for brunch. As they waited in the living room for Andy to finish getting dressed, which was taking longer than usual, he finally came downstairs in a mismatched outfit.

They laughed, thinking it was a joke, especially when Andy held his hands out and asked, "Does this match?"

With a smile, Laurie suggested that he go back upstairs and either change the pants or the shirt, and gave him ideas of which clothes in his closet would work.

Forty minutes later, Andy came back downstairs in the same outfit. The kids looked at him and said, "Dad, you're wearing the same thing!" But Andy had no recollection. Laurie had the kids wait downstairs when she went to the bedroom with Andy.

"I said, 'Honey, what happened?' And he said, 'Well, I took off my clothes and I guess I put them back on, right?' At that moment I knew there was something bigger than stress causing the cognitive changes. I knew we needed to have more assessments done to understand what was happening to Andy."

Laurie's concerns about Andy continued once he moved out. Memory challenges were affecting him personally and professionally. He would forget to pick up the girls from activities, get lost driving in familiar areas, and have difficulty using the TV remote control or opening the car door and using the seat belt. At work, Andy arrived late, missed meetings, did not consistently reply to emails, and frequently misplaced files. His partners began to question his competency. It was at this point that a more thorough diagnostic workup was done. Following a Beta Amyloid PET scan and spinal tap, a diagnosis of Young-Onset Alzheimer's Disease was given.

One of the most painful parts of this journey for everyone was that Andy met and spent time with individuals who noticed his cognitive decline and took advantage of him. On one occasion Laurie received a call from the local bank manager who was suspicious of a large withdrawal Andy was trying to make from their joint account. Andy was accompanied by a woman with a suitcase, hiding her face. Thankfully the bank manager knew Andy well. He denied the request and called Laurie. When Laurie asked Andy later about the incident, he had no memory of it.

With Andy living separately, Laurie would only discover his poor judgment after the fact. While Andy and Laurie discussed him moving back into the family home for support and care, there were significant safety issues related to the people now in Andy's life. They agreed that it would be best for Andy to stay at his apartment with a full-time assistant. Andy's decision-making skills continued to decline and following a middle-of-the-night incident involving the police, Laurie initiated a discussion about his functioning.

"It was a very loving conversation. I said, "Honey, you are not safe anymore. We need to look for a place where you can be safe and the girls can spend time with you and feel safe."

"Seeing that you were living apart, did he want you with him at the appointments?"

Laurie was firm with her response, having had to answer this hundreds of times over Andy's ordeal. "Oh yeah, we did everything together in terms of all the appointments. And it was interesting because one would think a couple being separated wouldn't, but that just was not our situation."

"Well, yes," I said, "That was what I was wondering."

Laurie smiled.

"Our situation was that we loved each other very much. There's been these challenges, but now let's figure it out together. That didn't change...that just didn't change."

"What was his reaction to the diagnosis?"

"Yeah, it was very interesting. The doctor came to get us in the waiting room, but he would not look me in the eye. I thought, this is not good. When we walked into the doctor's office, the brain scans were facing us. I had done enough research on these scans to know what to look for. The degree of blackness across the brain images confirmed my worst fear. I held Andy's hand as the doctor said the word— Young-Onset Alzheimer's Dementia. My heart sank but I didn't want to fill the room with my emotion. I wanted Andy to have the space to have his reactions. Andy held still and calmly said, 'Okay, what do we do?'"

Laurie paused, then pressed her lips together. "And that was that," she said, Laurie holding her hands open. "My heart was already sinking. There wasn't a lot of emotion at the time. Andy just said, 'Okay, what do we do?' The doctor said, 'Look, this is at the beginning. Hopefully, there will be more research on medication. These are the things you can focus on.' Hearing that made Andy feel more confident."

"So he was encouraged?"

"Yes. Right away, Andy got on board. He said, 'I'm going to be the first person who survives this. I'm going to be that person' and I wanted to support that for him."

Although Andy's enthusiasm was a good sign of his road towards an optimistic outlook, Laurie was more realistic about the eventual outcome of Andy's condition.

"At the same time, you're grieving, right? Because there's a part of me thinking, 'I know how research works. I know how slow things are. I know where things are in terms of the state of medication.' So there's this combination of wanting to support positivity but also grieve."

As time went on, Andy's optimism became unstoppable.

"Andy always, from the beginning of diagnosis until the end, was as positive as one could possibly be. And there were times where I just thought, 'If this were me, there is no way that I could do this.'"

I told Laurie I agreed with her. I don't know how I'd handle the diagnosis if I were in his shoes. It's also why I became so infatuated with the lives of the Optimistics. It's that constant belief of hope being the only way to survive dementia and be able to face each new day out of the darkness.

Laurie was always Andy's biggest champion and encouraged his definition of being a fighter for his disease. "He was always positive. He always said three things throughout his ordeal. First, 'I want to be the first person who survives this,' and then, 'I want to make the most of the time that I have.' However, it then shifted from, 'I'm going to be the first person to survive this' to 'I still want to be the first person that survived this.' He also was determined to make the most of what he had in terms of relationships with everyone."

The next promise Andy stood by had the most profound impact on Laurie and the kids. She continued to count off the list.

"And then the third thing he said, 'Is there anything I can do to help others?' So right away, we all got involved in the Alzheimer's Association."

Laurie recalled how infectious Andy's passion for raising awareness had become in the family. Laurie's youngest daughter even used Alzheimer's awareness as the backbone for a milestone in her own life.

"My younger one at the time was getting ready to be a Bat Mitzvah. She chose to do her Mitzvah project for Alzheimer's. She had always been a runner and decided that she was going to run 100 miles in a month as her Bat Mitzvah project. She would collect money and sponsors."

"Man, I couldn't run that in a year!" I replied.

"Well, she raised $6,000 for the Association. It was awesome! It was really, really awesome. We all got involved in the Walks and various things," Laurie said fondly.

Dementia's impact on Laurie's family didn't stop with the run. The kids took their passion to the big screen. "The girls did a national PSA that was shown in movie theaters." Then, Laurie wrinkled her nose, saying, "That was a little weird because a lot of people in the neighborhood didn't know, but then they saw the kids at the movies. From there, the kids also did a fundraising video for higher-level donors with the Alzheimer's Association."

Laurie continued to boast with pride about her daughters' work for Alzheimer's Dementia awareness, which showcased Andy's bravery in front of the public as well. Although

Andy was very open about his illness, representing the cause in person can be difficult as the disease progresses. Laurie worried that Andy's worsening condition may alter the confidence he fought so hard to keep. However, Andy did not disappoint.

"Andy decided that he wanted to speak at the Walks. So he did one, and then his functioning was decreasing, and he wasn't able to do more, but he still went to the Walks. That was his way of saying, 'I want to be the first person to survive. I want to be as positive as I can. I want my kids to see how one faces adversity with positivity. I want to see if there's a way of helping others.'"

Despite Andy's decline, he kept true to his three promises, no matter how hard each step became. I like to think that it's because of Laurie and the kids that Andy was able to keep his head up when so many times this disease will make you crawl away and hide. When there were times that Andy's positivity faltered, Laurie was there to hold him up. She tried not to take the credit for doing so, but without her, Andy's story would not have ended in a manner that the family could live with. Andy's daughters continue to be inspired by their father's optimism. Staying positive in the face of adversity and showing kindness and generosity to others who may be fighting silent battles of their own are themes they carry with them.

Amanda was fifteen, and Jaden was eleven when Andy was diagnosed. I told Laurie my kids are the same age now as hers were during that time. Knowing that kids have access to a world of knowledge via the internet, it was Amanda, in her big sister role, who decided to shield Jaden the most. She was adamant that her sister would be protected from some of the more challenging aspects of dementia. As much as Amanda wanted to safeguard her younger sister from the severity of Andy's condition, his cognitive and physical decline didn't allow him to do the same.

Laurie recalled the faces of her children during a night out for family dinner that pulled back the curtain on how badly dementia had taken over Andy's body.

"When was this? How long into Andy's condition?"

"This must have been maybe three years in," she said. "The first few years were just so challenging with all of the craziness. We all went out to dinner because we still celebrated holidays, birthdays, and all of that stuff together."

Laurie paused, remembering how that evening still impacted her children. "Andy couldn't cut his food," she said softly. "That was the moment that I saw it in Amanda's eyes. There was a shift from anger, disappointment, and hurt to more compassion. After that dinner, I remember her sharing, 'Mom, it's like working with one of my special needs kids.' When that resonated with her, all the other issues took a backseat. It was a turning point."

"It's incredible how those moments altered their lives in a positive way," I said. "How old is Amanda now?"

"She'll be twenty-seven in April."

While Amanda and Jaden grew up watching Andy's condition decline, Laurie, along with a huge community of family and friends, worked to provide them with as many joyful experiences as possible. This community helped guide them towards adulthood with wisdom and love. Andy remained involved in their lives as much as possible for as long as possible. In April of 2019, the family moved him closer to his brother Bradley, in Bloomington Indiana. Andy would be only five minutes away from his brother in a new dementia facility. This allowed for lots of visits and outings for Andy and Bradley and for their connection to grow, as well as great oversight of Andy's care. He was excited to be close to Bradley, but sad to leave Laurie and the girls. The night before the move—the first night of Passover—the family read a special prayer for Andy and shared their wishes for him. After dinner, they sat together and shared how they felt about the move, what they most appreciated about each other, and how much they would miss each other. Andy's language was limited by then, but he shared his love for his "three girls."

"There was consistent communication with Andy. It was all about the idea of we're this community taking care of Andy," Laurie said, pinching the air and flicking it out as if that thought of distance still had no place in her life. "Visits to Indiana, phone calls and zoom sessions were all a part of this new picture. Then COVID-19 hit and in-person visits from out of state relatives were no longer permitted. That made things very difficult. Bradley was allowed minimal visitation behind a plastic screen and Andy became more isolated."

COVID-19 limited visitations, but Bradley ensured that his brother would never be fully alone throughout his stay in Bloomington. Due to Andy's weakening body, he suffered a couple of falls at the living facility, which rattled his brittle frame. Between his battle with dementia, pandemic restrictions, and the falls, Andy's time was dissipating. Then, one day, Bradley received a call from the hospital that Andy's condition was coming down to the final stages. It was time to make the proper arrangements, so Bradley called Laurie. Because of pandemic restrictions, visitation was limited aside from Bradley. He set up video calls at the hospital to let everyone have a final private conversation with Andy.

"How long were those conversations?"

"My younger one had a lot to share, as she had just started college." Laurie said. "I think her call was close to an hour. I'm not sure how long Amanda's call was."

"What about you and Andy?"

"Andy and I had a lot of conversations before he left, and so my conversation at the end was not as long," she said, nodding.

"What was your last conversation with him about?" I asked, flipping my notebook over to a new page.

"My last conversation?" Laurie looked off to the side, remembering the hundreds of talks with Andy. "Well, there was a conversation when he wasn't conscious…" Laurie couldn't finish her sentence. She blinked and forced a smile as tears appeared behind her glasses. "So, my conversation was just talking to him."

Her voice was strained by the emotion when she remembered that day.

"It's okay," I said. "Take your time."

Through a crackled tone, Laurie said, "Mostly about the good stuff, because the bad stuff, I mean, truthfully, most of the bad stuff ended up being funny at some point because you just can't imagine. The conversation was really about years of goodness and how we've raised two really good, kind, compassionate, wise, and beautiful girls. They will take with them all of his goodness. And that he lived a good life. I'm just so appreciative of that and the time together. It was really just gratitude, respect, and love."

The final conversations care partners and loved ones have with people on their deathbeds are something no one can prepare for, as I've witnessed with others in this book. It's not a matter of what you say but that you choose to say it. Laurie took the opportunity to send Andy off with as much pride and dignity as anyone could ask for. Although he changed, Andy was still her husband and she still loved him.

During Andy's funeral, Laurie spoke to everyone. She shared with them, "Over the years many people have questioned me about why I stayed involved in Andy's care after our separation. The answer was always simple. I love him and we are family. That will never change. At this time of great loss, I stand here loving the man I married and divorced every bit as much as I did on our wedding day. It's a different, deeper, more knowing kind of love. But it is a complete love."

A year after Andy's passing, the family would get a chance to all come together for his stone-setting ceremony. In the Jewish religion, this ceremony is called the yahrtzeit and holds tremendous cultural meaning to Jewish families. At that time, friends and family gather around to witness the unveiling of the tombstone. For the months prior a smaller, stone nameplate was placed at Andy's grave. Laurie smiled wider than ever when talking about the yahrtzeit, remembering how special they made it for Andy.

"We were thinking about what to put on the headstone. And when the kids were little, on Friday nights, we would go around the table and talk about what we appreciated about each other during the week. When we started this tradition, Jaden was so young that she couldn't say appreciate. She said, 'I ap-eee-see-ate you' and it was the cutest thing ever," Laurie laughed.

I held up my hand and said, "Wait a second, how do you spell that? Because I know people will think I spelled it wrong when they read this."

"I agree. It's A-P-P-E-E-C-I-A-T-E. So at the bottom of the headstone, we put in quotes, "We appeeciate you." It was funny because the funeral home called me six times asking, 'Before we do this…' just to make sure I spelled it right and we did."

"That's so sweet, Laurie."

"That was the most accurate statement we could make about him, about his life, and our family."

Continuing to always put Andy above herself, Laurie thought about how their daughters recognized his legacy when he would no longer be around for them. She saved Andy's words of love for his daughters for their later years when his voice could no longer be heard.

"When we were going through this, for each kid's eighteenth birthday, I created a book for them with photos and a book of questions from Andy. I basically interviewed him. With Amanda, I would send him questions, and he would write back the answers. And then I put that together for her birthday. For Jaden, it was the same thing, but he couldn't write at the time, so we talked through the questions, and I wrote them down for him."

"Can I ask what it was about?"

Laurie nodded. "It was all about his feelings for them, what he wants for them. Lessons around relationships, money, and sex, like all the things that a parent would want to talk to their kids about. He also talked about how he felt about dementia and what he hopes people will remember him for. I think it's one of their prized possessions. They know that it was not Mom writing this for Dad. This was Dad's gift to them, in his words. Because he couldn't sign it himself, I made a copy of a previous signature from a card and then made a stamp for it. Now they each have that, and they have his thoughts, words, and feelings towards them."

I marveled at how well Laurie and Andy could co-parent and keep the love they each had alive in front of their children. It was a lesson of what it means to promise someone your heart and guide them through the bad times life will throw your way. It also made me think that Andy's overly optimistic viewpoint of dementia was the main contributor to allowing him to live as long as he did.

"You mentioned this earlier too, but with Andy, what he did was really about answering the question of 'How do you find the optimism?'"

"Absolutely," Laurie said firmly. "And he is the one that allowed us to hold on to that optimism. And God knows, like I said to you before, how he was able to muster that up, I do not know. I feel like that allowed our family to hold onto that throughout, and it only increased the love, respect, and appreciation for him."

"It was like his initial mission never stopped," I told her.

"Not at all," Laurie said, defiantly shaking her head. "Not. At. All. But he also had other things that brought him joy, which helped keep him optimistic."

"In which ways?"

"He was a scout for the Pittsburgh Pirates, so he loved baseball. He also loved Bruce Springsteen and traveling. He followed Bruce on a whole bunch of different tour locations. So yeah, baseball, Bruce, and traveling were his three passions," Laurie said, holding up three fingers. "When you think about that, all those things bring such joy—that helps someone maintain their optimism."

Before his burial, Laurie purchased a kippah with a Pittsburgh Pirates logo emblazoned on it. She placed it along with Andy's Bar Mitzvah tallit and a baseball the girls had signed and given to Andy one Father's Day in his casket. Laurie said it was something to show how much they loved Andy and always will.

CHAPTER SEVENTEEN

Lisa and Daniel

WATCH WITH WONDER

"She's the purpose in my life. Lisa, my daughters, and grandchildren—and my profession—are the purpose of my life"

When looking for others to connect with about their Young-Onset Dementia journey, Daniel was highly recommended as someone I should talk to from the beginning of this book. Deb kept asking me, "Did you talk to Daniel yet? Daniel is ready to talk to you" and so on. Getting our schedules to match was difficult. Daniel lives in El Salvador, is a full-time psychologist, and is a care partner for his wife, Lisa. Finally, we carved out a time when he was at the airport on the way to visit one of his three daughters, Gabriela, who lives in Panama.

The second Daniel popped onto the screen, he was smiling. He reminded me of a college professor with a compelling presence who can speak to hundreds of people at a time and command students' attention. Having lived in several countries since childhood, Daniel's accent is a unique mix of

Spanish, Hebrew, and English. His deep voice sounded like a radio announcer hosting a philosophy podcast.

It would be the first flight he'd taken without Lisa since her YOD diagnosis. I asked if he was excited for his flight, and he moved his body side to side as if to offer apparent nerves. "It's the first time I've left my wife behind."

"I don't like to leave her alone," he said with guilt. "I have four people right now that I hired to take care of Lisa. I don't have the memory care facility here in El Salvador, but I do have this group of people who support me in a very personalized kind of care."

I told Daniel he was fortunate to be able to provide such remarkable care for Lisa. It's hard for people to afford in-house care, let alone four people around the clock. Even though this is the only option due to his country's lack of proper care for people with dementia, he still has a choice to do less. Once you meet Daniel, you know quickly that he will never settle anything regarding Lisa. He made a firm decision from the time of her diagnosis that he would never leave her side regardless of how badly her condition developed.

"She will live forever in our home. We might downsize, I don't know, but she's now the main purpose in my life, you know? I don't know if that's called optimism?" Daniel said, shrugging his shoulders.

Dr. Daniel Guttfreund, PhD, is one of the most fascinating people I've ever met and one of the most traveled. He has lived in several American cities and Israel and now resides in El Salvador. His parents gave him a unique perspective about life and love when they discussed how they met.

"I'm a Jew by identity, very much in my roots. My mother was born in Romania but escaped to Berlin for a better life. Then, she escaped Berlin and went to Brazil. My father escaped Germany to El Salvador. He was looking for a Jewish wife and found her in Brazil."

He spoke about the struggles his parents endured to find one another and how, although Daniel fell in love with Lisa easily, their life together was anything but simple. Daniel and Lisa met in a clinical psychology PhD program in San Diego. Having so much in common and an immediate attraction, they began living together shortly after they started dating. They married in San Diego and then moved to Israel to start their family and continue their careers. Two years after arriving in Israel, the Gulf War had begun. Daniel had agreed with Lisa that Israel would be a trial period. Between wars, terrorist attacks and Lisa having her family very far away, Daniel realized it was getting too difficult for his family. He felt he had to honor Lisa's wishes and the trail period had to end. They had made a good life with their two daughters at this point, Maya and Gabriela, had to leave.

After going to many cities in the United States, Daniel and Lisa decided to move to El Salvador for a 1 year trial. Lisa could work part time to be able to be home and care for Maya and Gabriela, could be closer to her family. Daniel was there to try to look after the things his father left behind in El Salvador during the war in the eighties.

"We have three daughters, Maya and Gabriela, then Ilana was born in El Salvador. Lisa was able to be with the girls when they grew up, but she later worked. She was a psychologist for the Peace Corps volunteers in El Salvador and became the Head Of Counseling for the American School in El Salvador."

As two well-respected psychologists in El Salvador, they became popular among various circles in the medical community. Lisa survived breast cancer, but it was a precursor to her cognitive decline. As her cognitive condition worsened, she and Daniel discussed having her step down from certain roles. It was the American School that first approached her to resign. As an educational institution, they couldn't take the risk of having her work with the students in her unchecked condition.

Daniel remembers how that day affected Lisa. "She had no awareness. She was agitated and that's when it was very clear something more serious was happening."

In 2018, at the age of fifty-seven, Lisa was diagnosed with mild cognitive impairment—the first step to her YOD battle. The concept of having dementia at her age was something Lisa could not handle. Daniel noticed her normal personality began to turn dark as a result.

"Lisa had always been a very positive woman, and it almost went through one ear and went through the other. She didn't want to hear it. She was sort of more angry about why we were testing her. She has been in denial the whole time. A few years ago, we questioned whether we should be clearer about it, but we decided no. She's going to forget by the next day anyway. What's the point?"

If Daniel sounds defeated in having to throw his hands up about discussing Lisa's condition with her, he's nowhere close to it—he was at one point. There are moments when he cries in his hands alone, but he manages to speak openly to his clients of wife's Alzheimer's. Daniel is not a quitter. I commended him for keeping his emotions in check around his wife.

"She's now in stage six," Daniel said, looking at the side of our screen. He took a moment and told me, "I am the only person she fully recognizes."

The concerns about Lisa's memory towards others around her affect how she communicates, which is one of the things that Daniel misses most. "It's just having the person who was loving, intelligent, beyond bright, a real thinker, a polished person, and now that communication part is no longer."

Daniel's three daughters also feel the brunt of Lisa's condition and have to come to terms with her current identity and inability to communicate. The daughters all do their best to keep track of Lisa's progress, even when it's too hard to manage. With Maya living in London and Gabriela in Panama, Ilana is the only one close to home. Despite having a busy life, Maya and Gabriela still call every day. "Sometimes, Maya says she had a great talk with Lisa. And sometimes not."

As the closest daughter in proximity, she was the first to see Lisa's condition in real-time. Ilana told her father, "She's no longer the mother we knew." Daniel said, "Another example was when a neuropsychiatrist did an evaluation a month ago. He asked, 'Who's the person to your left?' It was our daughter, but Lisa said, 'It's my sister.'"

Even though Lisa can't remember her children, all of Daniel's daughters have a way of connecting with her. "With Ilana, they get into bed and watch movies and cuddle. Maya lives in London so she also tries to call. I think because she's so far away she was the one that struggled more and wanted to, from far away, to serve," Daniel said. "She wants to help and ask questions to the neuropsychiatric."

Daniel said spending time with Lisa in bed with Ilana was one of Lisa's favorite things. They'd lay under the blankets and watch the movie *Wonder* on repeat. Daniel told me it seemed to be the one movie Lisa had insisted on watching, which relaxed her mind. Even if Ilana isn't over, Daniel will still play the movie for her. Sometimes, he watches with Lisa; other times, he simply watches Lisa.

"What goes through your mind as you're watching her?"

"I used to love to watch her laugh. She was always a big laugher at slapstick, which I hated. But I laughed because she loved it. I have several recordings of her laughing—and I miss those laughs. There are a few sweet moments when she will say, 'I love you,' and I say, 'I love you too.' But for the rest of the days, she's walking around unhappy and agitated."

Between the medication to calm her emotions and the erratic behavior this disease torments its victims with, any sign of joy in Lisa brings immense satisfaction to Daniel. When Daniel was looking for support groups, he fell into a similar situation as other men, with not having male care partners to turn to. Finally, through various channels, he met others who became familiar faces to confide in.

"I find that dynamic you have with other guys in a group to be something very unique," I told Daniel. "Whether or not men are willing to or *can* be a care partner needs to be shared with the wider care partner community."

"It was hard to find an actual support group," he said "I was even thinking I needed to start my own support group for guys in my situation. Everything is about women care-takers. I posted on social media about anybody who wants to join a group on my forum. Eventually I connected to another group of men.

"How was that connection?"

"First, it was very large. Half of the men already had their wives in memory care facilities, while half of us did not. It's a whole different ball game. Then most of the men with wives in memory care facilities were already dating somebody."

Daniel wasn't looking to start dating again. Even in theory, it was an awkward conversation for him to have. Still, men helping other male care partners is a powerful movement that Daniel has benefited from over the years.

"What do you find that has been one of your biggest take-aways from that group? And how do you look at dementia as a care partner?"

Daniel shifted in his airport lounge seat, then rubbed his forehead, moving his thin eyeglasses off his nose. I could feel the emotion on his lips.

"What can I tell you, Richie, it's tough. And I would say it's cruel to the family members. Most days, I try to focus on my work and what I have to do, and then I come and start to be gentle and loving to my wife. But it's hard, you know, to be in a position where I come back for the whole day and then start a routine abating her."

The productive conversations Daniel and Lisa have today are minimal. He takes the wins where he can get them, which usually come in the form of humor. Daniel will tease Lisa that she doesn't love him. Lisa says she definitely does, only to have Daniel reply, "Oh, Lisa, you're a liar, liar, pants on fire." He does this knowing it will bring a smile to her face. When she says, "I love you," to Daniel, it's a painful reminder of the decades they had together before YOD. It also makes him cherish each time she says those three words, knowing one day that, her voice will likely disappear as a side effect of the disease.

"That's like the level of communication of trying to bond, you know, a little bit of that humor. I can't talk about the past. She doesn't remember."

"Does she ever ask about the past?"

"No, no. Actually, we were asking one of the helpers if she could start going through the thousands of pictures we had in a box, and then maybe Lisa would get involved, but it distressed her."

"Do you think she was missing it, or did she just not like that she didn't know the connection?"

Daniel heard photographs help individuals with dementia connect with people in their lives. He didn't want to give into Lisa's gripes and tried his humorous tactics to sway her frustration.

"I tried, but she didn't enjoy it. For example, I found a picture of her first boyfriend, who was seventeen, and I said, 'Look at this guy, your first boyfriend. God, what did you see in him? He's fat and ugly. Vince was more handsome.' But she just didn't connect, you know?"

Sometimes. Lisa would humor him in his friendly ways to make her comfortable, but other times, Lisa would be adamant about something out of her control.

"I lost her in Dulles Airport once. I sat in the chairs in front of the bathroom when we were flying to London, and for a few seconds, I looked at my phone. I didn't see her come out; I was right in front, and she just veered to the left. I found her ten gates later, looking for me."

On another occasion, Lisa mistook cockroach spray for sunscreen and rubbed dangerous chemicals all over her body. Daniel realized then that he had to lock things up and out of her reach. Daniel and his team of caregivers work around the clock to keep her safe and calm at home and at peace at night. As a doctor with a packed schedule, he is usually too exhausted to enjoy anything outside of the house by the time he gets home. His first concern is that Lisa has showered, is in bed, and is getting enough rest. Usually, he'll manage a game of chess or two and then find himself fast asleep shortly after. This is Daniel's new normal, a constant reminder of the two lives of Lisa he has lived.

"You mentioned that the girls miss their confidant in Lisa, the person they could talk to. What's the biggest thing you're missing right now from Lisa?"

Daniel's broad chest sighed. "Richie, I think the biggest thing is that she was such a big supporter of important issues and causes. In my life, she was a very non-judgmental person. And not being able to have a conversation with her..." Daniel is a warm person with a big heart, which he leaves open to everyone. When I heard him talk about what he missed, I hoped he would still find the energy to keep moving forward.

I asked him, "Does that affect your optimism? How do you remain optimistic, or even do you? And if you don't, that's fine too."

The question caused Daniel to press his lips tightly.

At that moment, I saw a man who had lived many lives through dementia. Someone in his position is owed the right to be both positive and negative when it comes to optimism, each without judgment. He's done it all. His highs of seeing how his daughters have taken on a maternal role to their mother have been startling for Daniel to witness. He has also seen through reaching out to others in his position he's not alone in his care partner role. The doctor in him knows he must advocate for others, no matter how hard discussing Lisa can feel. Then again, the darkness of this disease is a monstrous challenge for the strongest of wills to remain optimistic.

"I would say—I'm not sure it's optimism," Daniel said softly. "But, I try to be somebody who is not afraid to speak about this. I'm very vocal about this. I've been on the radio station and I make it a part of the narrative with my clients."

Of all the things he has to manage in his life, his work is a close secondary focus, as if on a mission to cure others of their pain in their battles.

"I just want my patients to be aware that's part of my life. I integrate this into my real life. The fact that I'm saying, 'I'm here focusing on you,' and I don't think they have felt in any shape or form that I'm not there in the same way. It's almost amazing how they don't even ask anymore. I might say, look, there's a little situation going on with my wife, so I might be interrupted by my assistant because something's going on. I'm not optimistic about the prognosis, obviously, but I am proud that she's still very active."

I told Daniel that the little wins could be gigantic regarding dementia. He shrugged his shoulders to close out his answer. When I returned to my notes, I underlined, circled, and asterisked the image of Lisa in bed watching *Wonder* on repeat. I remember when I took both of my kids to see the movie about a kid named Auggie who looked different on the outside from everyone else. I wanted them to appreciate what it's like to be different. Underneath, however, we're all looking for love, understanding, and companionship despite our insecurities that sometimes make life a struggle. For Lisa—as with others living with dementia—it's hard for them to express what they're truly feeling or thinking. Similar to the world around Auggie, no one outside of his shoes will ever truly know what it's like to be him.

I rewatched *Wonder* again, and one scene stuck out to me. One day after school, Auggie is in his room crying over his best friend who had betrayed him by using his appearance as a punchline to impress other kids in the class on Halloween.

Auggie refuses to trick-or-treat that night since he is so upset. His parents wanted to help, but he wouldn't listen. Then, his sister, offers to talk to him for them. As she tries to consult her brother, it's clear that today was unlike others.

He tells her that no one understands what it's like to be him. That he feels trapped and cornered by the negative treatment he must endure every day. His sister says she has bad days, too.

He fires back that no one's bad day could remotely compare to one his own. However, when his sister tells a story of her own best friend betraying her, it's clear that there is in fact someone who could understand his pain. She tells her brother that sometimes best friends come and go but the love of your family will never leave your side. It's in that belief that the two of them realize they'll never be alone, even when they feel the world around them is slipping away

In that scene, I saw Daniel and Lisa. Not only does *Wonder* teach the world about the sensitivity of others, but it also shows the struggle of living in a world where not everyone will accept you, just as dementia has done for Lisa. There will be bullies in life who challenge your confidence and dissect your insecurities, exposing them as damaged. Lisa's disease has done just that.

Lisa is fortunate to have a good network of people who will still take her to lunch, come over for coffee, and treat her as the woman she always was to them. The obvious doesn't have to be said to point out that Lisa has changed, yet bonds don't have to.

Lastly, the outside world is scary for people like Lisa who have to watch days go past them, too unsettled to capture moments as they speed past without notice.

After Daniel returned from his trip to Panama, we spoke again to continue his story. His smiling face popped up on the screen. "Shabbat Shalom!" he said.

"Yes! Gut Shabbes," I replied.

"How was Panama?"

"It was good. I had a great time with my family, and we got some things done that needed to be done."

"Speaking of family, I was hoping to hear more about how you and Lisa met."

In our first meeting, Daniel discussed how he and Lisa got together, but as I learned more about Dr. Daniel, I wanted to uncover deeper details of their love story.

"Okay, so the funny part is I had just come back from going back to Israel for two months and I had deeply fallen in love with an Israeli girl."

"You were with someone already?"

"Yes, in Israel. I was twenty-two and doing my extra year; Lisa was doing her first year. We started studying together and then went to Dollar Night movies on Wednesday nights. She kept insisting, saying, 'Why can't we take this further?' But again, I was in love with Amit in Israel."

Being 7,500 miles away and young, Daniel and Amit eventually broke up, and his relationship with Lisa flourished. They kept on studying together, becoming closer as friends, and a natural romance developed from there. Always a proper gentleman, Daniel insisted on meeting her mother since his intentions were more serious. Lisa, however, did not want to present him to her mother.

"I said, that's ridiculous! See, her mother was sort of a quirky lady. I've always thought of how I chose somebody so American and an American like Lisa chose this guy from all over the place," Daniel joked. "But yes, we moved in together a year later to a very beautiful offshoot community in San Diego before wanting to move to Israel."

"I imagine the conversation about moving across the globe was an interesting one? That kind of takes things to another level."

"Yeah, when I asked her to come to Israel to marry, she said, 'Honey, if I go to Israel, I'm already married. And if I don't like it there, we're leaving.' So, we got married and that's what happened."

While Daniel was talking, he occasionally looked off-screen at the door, asking, "Lisa? Lisa, are you there?" and then returning to talking. This time, however, he heard a large bang.

"Hold on," he said.

I could hear his muffled voice off-camera. Then he reappeared on screen again. "That was Lisa. I thought she needed something."

"No worries. You can go if you need to?"

"Oh no, it's fine. Maybe you would like to meet her?"

"Lisa? Yes! I mean, if that's okay?"

"Of course. Here, I'll take you with me."

Daniel brought me over to Lisa via the laptop screen.

"Lisa, I want you to meet somebody," and he points me in Lisa's direction. "This is Richie."

Lisa was all smiles when she saw me which gave me chills. Based on what Daniel was telling me, I didn't know what to expect. I assumed she would have been rather timid; however, Lisa was bubbly and energetic. She looked healthy, happy, and comfortable. Her hair was brushed in place and she even had a delicate tan. I would never have guessed her condition if I didn't know.

"Hi, Lisa. Good to see you."

She waved to me, "Hello. Thank you."

Daniel touched her arm while holding the computer with the other. "He's a friend who lives in the States. He's a writer."

Lisa's eyes lit up.

"He's also Jewish," Daniel added.

"Shabbat Shalom," I said.

"Shabbat Shalom," Lisa sang back.

Daniel turned the computer back towards his office and said to Lisa, "All right, so we'll let you go."

"Thank you, Daniel. She looks great," I said reassuringly.

"Yeah, that's when you see her like this, and she's very good. She makes you think that she knows you and is good to see you, but then two minutes later, something else can be happening."

Understanding that Lisa's condition is more strenuous than comforting, I saw a woman with a tremendous amount of life in her and reminded Daniel the same thing. We started to talk again about Lisa's next steps. Daniel already said she would remain in the house until her final days. But for Daniel, life after Lisa will occur without his control.

"Have you started to piece together what you think your life is going to be like when Lisa is gone?"

Daniel replied immediately. "No," he replied firmly. "I'm not going there."

The husband and provider in Daniel wants to make sure his wife never goes without the slightest need she may require, as if every little step will buy him one more moment with Lisa. Then, the veteran doctor side of Daniel knows enough about science and medicine to realize the clock is working against his efforts to pause the gentle moments he can celebrate. I told Daniel I like to think there is room for pure optimism and fact-based reality, even if one tends to overshadow the other, casting an uncertain future regarding their lives together.

Although Daniel doesn't like to think about years down the road without Lisa, he is unfortunately learning the separation between who she was and who she is today. When

Daniel talked about the effort he had put into connecting with Lisa, he faced the fact she would never again return it in the same manner.

"Richie, it's a feeling like you're in a relationship with somebody who is no longer there."

Throughout this book, I discuss the choices care partners and people with dementia have when it comes to handling the disease: stay in the darkness or find the light. To Daniel and his daughters' credit, I believe Lisa found that light because they showed her how.

Today, Daniel still runs his therapy practice, counsels others hurting like him, travels to see his daughters, and speaks with anyone who needs an empathetic ear. As he does every day, despite the professional, financial, and emotional exhaustion his life brings, Daniel cherishes the time he has left with Lisa and seeing the love of his life resting in their bed. Although he knows it won't be this way forever and the days are never long enough, Daniel will ensure that Lisa is just as loved as ever until her final breath. In that belief, there's a beautiful sense of wonder.

CHAPTER EIGHTEEN

Wendy and Doug
MIDNIGHT JOURNALS

*"If you can live a life to love a life, then Life itself has been worth living". —*Doug

"One thing I do know—I know where I'm heading. I know it's not going to get easier."

I received Doug's information from Deb as someone I should speak to for this book. The only information I had was his wife was diagnosed with a rare form of dementia and Doug had a rather unique way of coping. We met on video call while Doug sat in his car outside of a work appointment. He's had a very successful business for decade but downsized his career after Wendy's diagnosis. He stopped traveling for work and engages in limited sports and activities where Wendy can join him. Doug says finding a distraction is important or dementia would overtake their lives.

Doug and Wendy began their lives together at eighteen, while freshmen in college, and never looked back. Doug refers to their lives as fast-tracked. They married after college and had three boys. Doug started a business, which Wendy helped grow, and both turned it into a rewarding operation. Life was good, and as Doug said, he always felt that something higher helped put his dream life together.

Then things changed.

"It started with Wendy's operation for a hysterectomy. She was put to sleep, and they couldn't wake her up. The doctors came out and were panicking. What's going on?"

Doug described the frenzy of Wendy's state as a race to restore Wendy from an unknown coma. "We're trying to wake her up. We're putting smelling salt stuff underneath her nose."

It took an hour and a half to revive Wendy, and after, she would never be the same. Shortly after Wendy's operation, Doug noticed slight changes in her speech. She missed or mispronounced words she usually handled with ease. With no inclination that could be anything more than minor hiccups, Doug and Wendy laughed it off. Her verbal fumbles became a running joke at first. However, as time passed, Wendy seemed to struggle physically with communication. Six months after her surgery, her condition became more challenging, and as Doug said, "It wasn't so funny anymore."

With no direct cause for her declining speech, Doug looked to a nutritionist, thinking it may be a dietary issue that morphed into verbal abnormalities. After that, Wendy's condition wasn't resolved, so they searched for a wider array of specialists to help make sense of her behavior. Doug read an article about Lyme Disease. It seemed similar to what Wendy was experiencing, so Doug explored that path. Through various procedures and a Lyme specialist for another six months, they wrote that off as well. At that point, nothing had helped to revert Wendy's speech to where it had been before the surgery. Failing to find answers, Doug contacted a speech therapist to try to retrain or correct her speech.

Doug came across a top specialist at Loyola University in Baltimore who was highly recommended. After an initial session with the therapist, she told them to get Wendy checked out for something other than Lyme Disease and speech.

"Great, back to square one," Doug thought.

Determined to uncover the mystery behind her predicament, they found a specialist at the prestigious Johns Hopkins University. At Hopkins, Wendy would be diagnosed with Semantic Variant Primary Progressive Aphasia (svPPA). PPA alters someone's speech and understanding of words, causing difficulty in identifying faces and objects. Finally, they had a title for her condition; one they could now follow, track, and help resolve. Wendy continued to see the specialist, and eventually, the visits led to her final diagnosis: Semantic Dementia.

"We were shocked! We didn't know what PPA was or what was going on. Wendy was extremely upset about that, and I was really upset too. One of the issues that they tell you right from the onset is there's nothing we can do about it."

Doug wouldn't accept "nothing" as the only answer.

Continuing Doug's tour of academia, his research pointed him to Georgetown University, for a different speech therapy. Those sessions were more extreme than what Wendy endured at Loyola, which included more MRIs to track her progress. Sadly, that did not work either. Doug felt lost, misguided down a path of arrows pointing him down dead-end roads.

With every therapist interaction, Doug heard the voice of her doctors in his head, reminding him that this would likely only get worse. Determined for a change, Doug continued to entertain any resources to slow down or reverse Wendy's condition. He read about therapies, made calls, and took her to various doctor appointments, but nothing worked.

"It was just prolonging. Eventually, words disappeared from her vocabulary, but it was an interesting situation moving along. Then, we thought the process was, well, who else could we see who could give us more information? At least so that we could tell our kids that they might not be so susceptible to getting it themselves."

Doug's work days were overtaken by obsessing over researching to see if anyone could offer their expertise. He had already visited some of the top medical facilities on the East Coast and still came up empty. He talked to friends whose parents went through Alzheimer's Dementia, took advice from their other doctors, and reached out to people he saw on TV in interviews. Anyone, anywhere. Eventually, someone pointed him to the National Institute of Health (NIH). He enrolled her in a series of tests they were offering for those with dementia. Not only did the sessions not work for Wendy, but they resulted in a severely traumatic experience for her. At NIH, she underwent spinal taps which brought on panic attacks and a nervous breakdown. Doug wanted to take Wendy's pain as his own, even feeling guilty for putting her through the trials. Doug questioned how far he would have to go to find the medical answers to what would make Wendy's life more manageable.

"What else do I need to do?"

To make matters worse, Wendy would be re-diagnosed with PPA Mixed Variant rather than the Semantic Variant. Doug threw his hands up. At this point, he had given up on the labels on his wife. Instead, he focused on how to make her life more accessible and more manageable and like many other care partners, a way towards a more comfortable normal. Doug also needed to recharge his mental comfort. He needed an outlet to express himself, even if no one was listening. Maybe then he would find answers through the darkness.

Doug doesn't remember how his mind pointed him to writing, but he began journaling daily to keep track of Wendy's progress and relieve some of his aggravations. The process was therapeutic and became a way to speak with his inner dialogue that kept fighting for his time.

"I don't know where the suggestion for journaling came from, but I did it for several reasons. Number one, to document and help me understand where we were in this process. And number two, perhaps have something to reflect on so I could get an idea of what was happening. You know, what was going on a year ago? What was going on two years ago?"

As someone who puts pen to paper daily, I was happy Doug used his writing to gather his feelings. Since Doug seemed to enjoy the process, I assumed writing was something he was familiar with; however, Doug never perceived himself as a writer. Not only that, he never looked at his journaling—at first—as working on a story to chronicle his moods daily.

As a result, a particular healing process emerged—and at the most unique times.

"I needed to get stuff out. I'd be writing at times when things were tough, and whether it was to talk to somebody or to write it down, it was easier for me to write it down. A lot of times, you wake up at two in the morning, and you've got all these thoughts. What do you do?" Doug said, shrugging his shoulders.

Rather than allow his negative thoughts to consume him, Doug answered the agony he felt at that moment, regardless of the time. Nighttime let him fully embrace his writing since Wendy would be asleep, and Doug knew she was safe. He also didn't want Wendy to see the expressions on his face and the toll on his body that her disease had caused him. That was the darkness of this disease, and Doug could not allow that part to take over. Instead, he used the darkness of night as his confidant rather than a foe.

"Now, I journal whenever I feel like it, you know? It helped me to understand that this is something that's out of my control. I would be able to look at what I wrote and say, even if it's something that wasn't, you know, totally optimistic, I'd be able to look at it and say to myself, 'Well, I get why you wrote that'."

Doug's journaling also encouraged him to engage with others in his position. He went to groups and heard others talk about their issues. Although it proved he was not alone, he never felt truly connected to those in the groups. Yes, others had it bad–awful at most times–but Doug didn't want to focus on the negative. Instead, Doug wanted to concentrate on what good could be done. Focusing on the sadness of this disease was a given, and Doug had been through enough. This disease will not change as your mind leans towards the positive. Yet, the attitude towards finding optimism in the smallest light passing through the days seems the only solution to survival.

Doug rallied behind that belief and poured it into his journaling. From his phone, he offered to read one of his latest entries. "I wrote this today to myself."

Wendy is starting to get more and more confused.

She cannot understand anything she says anymore.

I sense she knows she is going downhill.

The disease is eating away at her very existence.

What a tragedy to sit by and watch the fall in slow motion.

My heart is heavy and I feel so sad.

I cannot describe my life any better than dealing with daily loss and no hope.

Doug placed his phone back into his lap. We both took a breath. I held back tears.

At that moment, I saw Doug's late-night sessions, trying to make sense of his situation. I saw the man restless, yet tired and hopeful while hopeless. It was his life behind the tough exterior of a man fighting a battle that only he can understand. His armor is thick because he tries to take on as much pain as he can from Wendy and his family, but even the toughest shell can crack under immense pressure. They say the pen is mightier, but the writer's heart wielding the ink controls the narrative on the page. Doug's journals are not only his thoughts but proof of his journey and a reminder not to give up on his cause.

"I'll read what I said to myself on particularly rough days when I'm not so positive and when I can't endure. I like to remind myself that my track record for getting through bad days so far is a hundred percent. That's pretty good."

I was slowly nodding along to his words in a trance.

Then he added, "And that's the message of hope. There I was dipping, and then I grabbed myself by the shoulders and pulled myself upright."

Doug surely knows how to capture his voice and express his emotions for a man who doesn't call himself a writer. He looked at me to see what I thought. He was connecting with me as an outsider looking in.

I told Doug that I admired his consistency and strength in reminding himself that he could not allow his mind to spend too much time in the darkness. Through his journals, he found a way out. Most people, myself included, could not confidently say they could do the same.

"What I was trying to tell you, Richie, is I'm fighting it all the time. There are two things you can't do. If you have a period where you're going to break down, one of the things to do is to write down what you're thinking. Then, once you're finished writing that down, it doesn't have to be a long period, but think about how I want to handle this."

Curious, I asked Doug if his two-step approach was mirrored across the board in his family.

"How have your kids reacted? Do they have the same mentality as you do about this?"

Doug has three boys, all of whom have families and adult lives. He knows they want to be there for Wendy, but Doug also knows they can do only so much. His biggest fear as a father was to feel like he would enhance the boys' level of worry and distract them from their families. He wants to protect his kids from the pain Doug wrestles daily, yet at the same time, he doesn't want his children at a distance either. It's a balancing act, he admitted. One where the father is the safeguard from harm and must continue that role, even though they are all grown men with fatherly roles.

"This thing can affect the performance of what your kids are trying to achieve in life. I don't want to do anything to affect my children's opportunity to perform at a peak while they're trying to raise kids and build their lives."

This mental ping-pong match was more emotional for Doug during their fortieth wedding anniversary. The date was always a happy time before her illness. Now the date was something he saw in the distance, fearing she may not make it to many more. Doug wanted to make the milestone as normal as possible for his children, even though there would be no party to toast their love as there had been in years past.

As Doug's social calendar became nonexistent, their inner circle siloed to their house, with Doug's home-cooked meals for Wendy. He admits that cooking was never his thing but with dementia, becoming a chef is a welcomed role compared to others he has had to take on or attempt.

Still, Doug finds the positive about their situation and Wendy's condition compared to how bad it is for others. He told me about a dear friend of his with MS who can't walk and is confined to a wheelchair. While Wendy's mental state is a disability, she can still go for walks, take trips to the mall, dine out, and enjoy the beach. His friend cannot. Learning to appreciate life more has been a gift that Doug did not expect.

Reminding him of the good fortune of still having Wendy around, he takes her on as many walks as he can.

From having kids around to being outside with one another to pointing out the importance of their incredible anniversary, Doug does his best not to focus on what Wendy can't do anymore. He also chooses to provide an attempt at normalcy for Wendy despite the times that cruelly remind him her situation is anything but that.

"I still to this day, take her out on the golf course. To give you an example of where she is playing golf now, she was the club champion. Now she can't take the ball and put it on the ground. When I give her a club she doesn't know where to stand. If she finally finds the ball, she will hit it sideways."

There have been many reports of rare cases of people with dementia who had careers in the arts, especially where they'll remember a song, how to paint, or a dance that reflects their life before the disease. Doug isn't expecting Wendy to get a bolt of energy when she approaches the tee. He simply wants her to be around what she loves. At one point, Wendy's life was golf, yet seeing her revert to a toddler's ability on the course rips Doug apart. Regardless, he keeps doing it for Wendy, hoping for that rare moment when something will click. In the meantime, he learned to hide his emotions from her, even though she can't process his feelings.

"Richie, your heart hurts because you're sad. All I'm doing is trying to make her comfortable. But it's like throwing a heavy ball at your chest and how do you endure that feeling? Again, I write down how I'm feeling and then take a look at it."

With everything that Doug does to bring moments to Wendy, I wondered how he believes she sees it.

"How does she communicate with you now?" I asked.

Doug shook his head. "I used to be able to understand her from hand gestures, and maybe she could point something out to me. We've gotten past that. I don't understand her anymore. I make her think that I understand. And she'll stop talking."

The break in communication for care partners is one of the hardest aspects of the disease to accept. Not knowing how their partner feels about what they need or want, the care partner can lose hope quickly. Wendy's decline, especially in her communication, is a constant reminder that Doug's attempts to engage with her will only be met with blank stares. He recalled one of his journal entries when picturing Wendy's eyes meeting his with no acknowledgment.

"One thing I do know is I know where I'm heading. I know where, and it's not going to get easier."

"What do you mean when you say you know where you're heading?"

"Richie, I'm fortunate enough to have done fairly well in my business. Even though I had ended my business career—not the way I wanted to—by selling out to my business partner and reducing my work schedule, I dropped out of things I was involved with. I did it because this is what I wanted to do. And I'm going to take care of her until I can't take care of her anymore. Do I have a plan? Yeah, I have a plan."

I don't know what Doug's long-term plan is for Wendy. For now, the best way he knows to make her comfortable is by changing her scenery and keeping her active. This could be walking the golf course for as long as that lasts. Sometimes, they'll get take-out food or go to the restaurant. On occasion, it's just a drive.

"When you do things like that, how does she react? Do you think she knows it's something different?"

"Sometimes she reacts in a, you know, a way?"

Doug smiles even though Wendy can't, hoping she'll see that joy. He wants her to know he's okay with being by her side, no matter the condition.

"I wrote a list of every place that Wendy likes to go to eat and what she likes at those places."

Doug smiled, thinking about his list as if he was courting her when they began dating. He's a romantic. He still wants to win her over like they were in their twenties. He wasn't the only one involved in Wendy's trips either. At the beginning of her condition, their friends would ask what they could do and how to help. Overwhelmed with requests, Doug created a calendar for days Wendy could go out and then shared the link. Doug was excited to see her dance card filled with familiar faces in her life.

"I will share the chart with you sometime, Richie. I used it as my talking tool at first, you know. Everyone who asked, 'What can I do?' I'd share that calendar with them. And what I thought would happen is people would start calling up and saying, oh, I see Wendy's free here. During that same time, that's when I wrote the letter of all the things that she likes to do, where she likes to go, the restaurant likes, and the parks that she likes to go to."

Despite early attempts to take Wendy out, eventually, the calendar went unanswered.

"I thought that was the biggest disappointment of this whole thing. I thought that all these friends that we had would be stepping up and jumping in to help out. There was a couple that did for a little bit. It soon became, you know... it was sad. It became something that nobody was referring to anymore."

Doug shrugged his shoulders in a "that was that" manner.

"I think you realize who the people are who really matter in the end and who you can or want to be around. The thought process of talking yourself out of a negative and making your life more positive is something you have to do. Otherwise, it would just drag you down. It's very simple: is the glass half empty or half full? When you're a caregiver, you don't have a choice but to be half full, or three-quarters full at least."

I stop him. "Even three-quarters is a lot, Doug," I said. "I think that's better than most."

"It sounds easier said than done," he replied knowingly. "And I say three-quarters full because I don't want to bring my wife down. She's already dealing with a bad situation. I want to make her happy. I think the thought process is, when I hear about optimists, I kind of chuckle about them because it's just—you don't have a choice."

I had to disagree with Doug here because he does have a choice. Everyone can choose to point their lives in any direction, regardless of how severe their issues may affect their well-being. That point alone is the meaning of the Optimistics.

—How do you stay optimistic when everything seems hopeless?

—How can you keep your head above water when the darkness

takes over your body?

—How can you explain to others who aren't in your position
what it feels like to burrow into a small hole of silence?

I challenged Doug about how he decided to choose optimism. Doug's answer was writing. I told him that writing cured me as well.

"If you want to combat this in the way you need to, you have to be an optimist and look at things in a way that makes you the most capable of dealing positively with the situation for you and your wife or husband or whoever it might be. I will have a moment where I'll write down something. You write it down, and you look at it, and you say, okay, well, is that what you want to dwell on?"

Today, Doug continues to operate his business while he cares for Wendy. The provider in him will never slow down, nor will he quit looking for more answers from anyone who can offer solutions.

"Even today, with few words left and no ability to take care of herself, Wendy still is beautiful, has maintained some empathy, a warm smile. She is loved by all her caregivers and those who have chosen to stay engaged," Doug said. "I'm not sure what the future holds, but for now, I will take that as a positive!"

He still encourages others to spend time with her while they can; however, Doug is more than happy to take every minute of every date with Wendy for himself.

CHAPTER NINETEEN

Looking Back and Walking Forward

When I first decided to write a memoir, a fellow author friend told me, "Memoirs only work if the events you're discussing changed you in the end."

"Okay. Understood," I said. Then, after my first YES group meeting, I told him, "I'm changed."

He laughed. "No, through the process, not after one day."

"I know," I replied. "But I'm telling you, I'm already a different person."

"Well, then," he said, humoring my excitement, "I can't wait to hear how you feel when the book is done."

He was right about this book's meaning developing over time, and he was also correct that I felt dramatically different when I completed *The Optmistics*. However, one aspect of my journey that derailed his theory is that there is no end for me with Optimistics. This book may be over, but the next step as an Optimist is nowhere close to being done. I still have work to do to honor the Optimistics and care partners worldwide. If Dennis taught me anything, it's that **time is important**.

Time can't be wasted, abused, or neglected, nor can I allow anyone to take time away from me. We own our time, but that only comes with agreeing to use it without regret.

At the beginning of this book, I talked about how no publisher understood that a book like this couldn't go through the standard publishing pipeline. I didn't have two years after the book was complete to share the Optimistics' stories, and neither did they. I saw them change their identities as Alzheimer's slowly pealed away at their clock. I knew the individuals I spoke to would be different when I completed this book, but I had no idea the harshness of that difference and how fast it would occur.

In Sarah's chapter, I watched her stories of optimism about her mother's health turn into the reality of her untimely death less than forty days later. During our interview, the concept of death was never on the table—there was only hope. Sarah knew her mother had less time than most people living with Alzheimer's but never thought the decline would be so rapid. She and her mother were victims of the way Alzheimer's will steal your plans and dissolve your perceptions of the future into a mere afterthought. Still, through all of that pain, Sarah could not allow herself to fall back into the darkness that this disease once held her captive. Her mother would not have wanted that. In her most challenging times, although her mother was gone, Sarah could still feel her mother's hand in hers.

Other care partners I met saw their spouses or parents leave their homes and move into assisted living facilities, knowing full well they would not return to their bedside. I listened to Michael describe the insufferable first night alone in over four decades without Carla. Daniel spoke openly about how Lisa was an entirely different person now. I watched the pain and frustration in Shannon's eyes when discussing how her mother's inability to appreciate Shannon's efforts was not a reflection of their love. In every situation, it was the disease that was speaking for those living with dementia and not the person their loved one knew before the disease took control.

A list of changes to my psyche I went through because of my interaction with the Optimistics deserves a sequel to fully illustrate how much the past two years turned my life around. However, from all the ways that everyone in this book affected my life, the most impactful message is that **time is important.** Those three words became the driving force out of personal darkness to believe in something greater than I ever imagined for this book. The bonds I've created with strangers showed me the importance of time spent and time left.

Like many adults working to achieve success, there is a race against time to reach "the top" for whatever purpose may be for them. When that happens, you can miss out on other aspects of life essential to true fulfillment. The idea of pushing myself towards a goal, despite my anxieties, has been a struggle for me my entire life. I've allowed myself to get lost in other's opinions rather than listening to myself or, at the very least, believing in myself enough to dismiss their negativity. I allowed those publishers to tell me this book wouldn't happen. When I think back to all the time I wasted focusing on doubts thrown at me by others about this book, I realize how much I missed.

As any writer will tell you, the process of the writing experience is different for every project, and the feelings during that time can be a complicated concept to handle. The notion that **time is important** seeped into every aspect of my day at times when I was least expecting it. I saw professional engagements that were solely one-sided by me take a back seat quicker than in the past because no amount of time would amount to anything fruitful. Friendships that seemed more work than pleasure went filed away, whereas the tight group that truly understood the meaning of dedication took a more significant place. With family, I became more emotional as time went by at a rate I thought I could govern. I took pictures of family moments and tried to be more present and take time to focus on patience over quick reactions. **Time is important** also triggered my brain for strangers I saw who may not have much time left either.

For instance, I recently took my family to a brunch restaurant to a Baltimore staple called Miss Shirley's Cafe, which has become my go-to birthday destination. While I filled my mouth with stacks of chocolate chip pancakes that resembled sofa pillows and an omelet the size of a football, I noticed two grandparents with their college-aged grandson a few tables away. The grandmother's hand shook slightly as she held her fork, and the grandfather hunched over his plate like someone trying to look closely at a laptop screen. They laughed and smiled as the boy talked about college life. He even offered to pay, but his grandfather patted his hand away. The boy hugged them goodbye when they were done and held his grandmother's hand out the door.

I have no idea who these people are, and I will likely never see them again, but I fell in love with their relationship because it was genuine and relatable. At that moment, I thought about other Optmistics with children and grandchildren who would look at a Sunday brunch with their loved ones on a random spring day as one of the greatest memories they had together. I also thought of that young man, years from now at his first "real job" getting a phone call from his parents one day about the passing of his brunch partners.

Repeatedly, I hid from the pressure I put on myself to share the Optimistics' journeys properly. The intense emotions I felt from hearing their stories were far beyond my initial preparation. I thought I would be the outsider looking in, but I quickly became invested like their family. We laughed together, cried as one, and thanked each other for sharing our vulnerabilities.

When I thought back to all the times my emotions caused me to take a break and put the pen down, I remembered the promises I made to the Optimistics' families. I had to train my mind to focus on the bonds I had with each Optimistic and their care partner, which was the fuel that allowed me to escape the emotions this book put on my body. I learned that although the shadows that stalked my confidence were shades brighter on its worst days than anything an Optimistic would go through. Realizing that if they could face their lives with gratitude, I could use their optimism to step forward each day.

The me *before* the Optimistics would have crumbled under the pressure of my anxiety toward ensuring I was on the right path, but then, I'd get help from someone rooting me on. I'd receive a text or email from Deb, who was a lifeline of encouragement in her belief in me, even to the point of tears at times. She would remind me of how this book will help change the lives of the Optimistics and how much the YOD community needs their voices heard. Every moment I spent with the Optimistics reinstalled the notion that the outcome of this book will create more awareness for people like them, who think they are alone with their condition. Their passion made it so I could never break, no matter how often my heart and soul bent through the storms.

Every day, the Optimists lose more of their lives than before but refuse to give up. Each doctor's appointment brings them another cocktail of hope. Despite knowing there is no cure in their lifetime, the Optimistics choose optimism over fear and hope over doubt. Without that mindset, time stops becoming essential but rather an admission that time has gotten the best of them.

I remember a group text exchange with Mike and Dennis. Referring to a time when Mike was having a rough moment, Dennis said, "I hope the last few weeks have been enjoyable in the daytime and pleasant at night, with better breathing and bright sunshine." His words were a reminder when you feel like time is slipping away and life is having its cruel way with you, take a moment to breathe in the present and wink back at the sun.

Although I still don't quite believe that everything happens for a reason (sorry, some things never change), I do believe in the power of timing. Because of the Optmistics, I learned the value of making every second matter because I have no idea what will happen tomorrow, let alone in the next hour. The Optimistics taught me to appreciate what's in front of me now and not ruin those moments by debating what roadblock will stop me in the future. Dennis, time is important, and hope—although difficult to see at times—is always there.

Optimism is not a right; it's a choice in which you can either embrace hope or embody doubt.

Thank You

From people behind the scenes to my champions who put themselves out there for me through this process, my thank-you list could go on forever.

First, to my wife and kids, who have the daunting task of admitting they know me and even related to me, it isn't always easy. Despite my weirdness, there isn't a single minute of my life that I don't have all of you on my mind. Every single thing I do is for you. I hope I made you proud.

To my wonderful editor and publisher at The Omnibus Publishing, Wendy Dean, who believed in me from day one. Handling my ADHD and wandering mind daily is what some may call challenging, and I'm grateful for your patience. When I called you about this book, the first thing you said was, "I'm in." With every word I typed, you kept that promise.

To Deb and the YES Foundation, this would NOT have happened without you. You cheered me on at full volume and continued to amaze me with your trust. What you're doing for the Alzheimer's community, especially in Baltimore, deserves all the attention in the world. When times got tough for me throughout this journey, Deb was always there to keep me motivated. Deb, you're the cornerman every fighter needs to battle Alzheimer's. This story is for you.

To the Alzheimer's Association of Maryland, your belief in me was an incredible honor. You are a resource for help and guidance through the world of Alzheimer's, and it's because of you that we will #EndAlz.

And finally, to all of my Optimistics, the only words that make sense are "I love you." I love you for letting me into your world. I love you for allowing me into your homes. I love you for your honesty. I love you for your self-belief and ability to step out of the darkness of Alzheimer's. And I love you for making me realize there is optimism in life, no matter how hard one's road may become. Most importantly, I love you for showing me how and why **time is important.**

RESOURCES AND SUPPORT

Call the Alzheimer's Association

If you're living with Alzheimer's or dementia, or care about someone who is, we're only a phone call away. The Alzheimer's Association 24/7 Helpline is staffed by experts who provide free, confidential information that includes resource lists, caregiving tips, care planning support, clinicial trial information, education programs and support groups. Don't wait for a crisis to call. We're here whenever you want to talk.

One call can make a difference.
24/7 Helpline: 800.272.3900

Visit alz.org

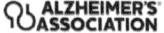

ABOUT YES!

YES!, Inc. (Young-onset dementia Education and Support) is a 501(c)(3) organization, established to address the under recognized and growing needs of the YOD (Young-Onset Dementia) community. A dementia diagnosis for those in their 40s, 50s, or 60s creates unique challenges not germane to older-onset dementias. YES! strives to bridge the gap between isolation and resources through emotional support and practical solutions for YOD-affected families. Fostering interpersonal connections and normalizing the often simultaneous sadness and humor of YOD is what propels the organization.

YES! facilitates nationwide virtual and local in-person support groups for care partners and their families, including high school youth and young adults. YES! also offers care provider retreats, field trips, and topic-focused resources, and empowers those diagnosed with YOD to seize opportunities for peer-to-peer engagement, such as the Optimistics.

All YES! team members have personal or professional experience with YOD, and whose passion and empathy permeates every facet of the organization. YES! has a resource relationship with the Alzheimer's Association, Greater Maryland Chapter, and works collaboratively with, University of Maryland School of Pharmacy, Johns Hopkins Medicine's FTD, and Young-Onset Dementias Clinic, as well other non-profits and support networks of other dementias commonly diagnosed in the sixty-five years-and-under age group.

More information about YES! can be found by visiting their website at https://www.yessupport.org.

Resources and Support

FOR PEOPLE WITH DEMENTIA AND THEIR CAREGIVERS

NATIONAL NONPROFIT ORGANIZATIONS:

Alzheimer's Association - https://www.alz.org/

Alzheimer's Foundation of America - https://alzfdn.org/

Lewy Body Dementia Association - https://www.lbda.org/

Lewy Body Dementia Resource Center - https://lewybodyresourcecenter.org/

Association for Frontotemporal Degeneration - https://www.theaftd.org/

National Task Group on Intellectual Disabilities and Dementia Practices - https://www.the-ntg.org/

LOCAL AND STATE GOVERNMENT OR TRIBAL SOCIAL SERVICES AND PROGRAMS:

Elder Care Locator -
https://eldercare.acl.gov/Public/Index.aspx

Indian Health Services - https://www.ihs.gov/

COMMUNITY RESOURCES

Faith-based organizations, check your local ministry

Your local Area Agency on Aging -
https://www.usaging.org/

Local chapters of the Alzheimer's Association
https://www.alz.org/local_resources/
find_your_local_chapter

For more information and to explore the links listed here, please visit the official website of the United States Government at the web address below:
https://www.alzheimers.gov/life-with-dementia/
find-local-services

Meet Richie Frieman

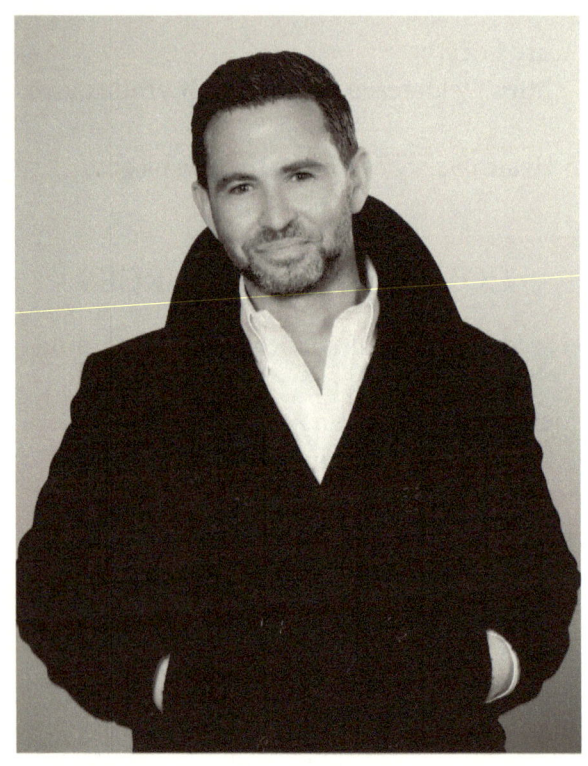

About Richie Frieman

St. Martin's Press and Macmillan Publishing dubbed Richie Frieman a "Modern Day Renaissance Man" due to a career that spans life as an author, illustrator, artist, etiquette expert Modern Manners Guy, entrepreneur, screenwriter, cartoonist, and even a champion professional wrestler. He is a #1 best-selling and award-winning author and illustrator of eight books in multiple genres, with work being sold worldwide.

Recently, Frieman was part of Kwame Alexander's pilot for his new TV show, "America's Next Great Author" and will be a part of the show's professional cast. Over the years, Frieman's success has landed him on media outlets across the globe, appearing live on numerous radio and TV shows, including MSNBC and FOX News Entertainment, and featured in Time Magazine, Money Magazine, Yahoo, Martha Stewart, Forbes Magazine, The Wall Street Journal, Entrepreneur Magazine, Huffington Post, Fast Company, USA Today, Publishers Weekly, Parade, Story Monsters Ink, and many more.

For more information, visit www.RichieFrieman.com.